Run and Smell the Roses

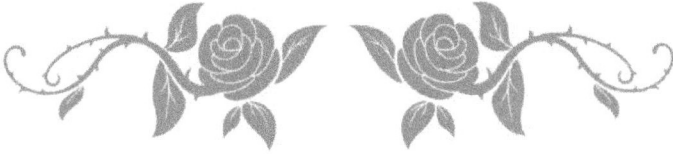

*Our Journey to Physical, Mental and Spiritual Transformation
Through Running*

Yolanda Diaz and Itarsha Payne

DCC Publishing, LLC.
dccpublishing@gmail.com

Yolanda and Itarsha can come to your live event. For information about special discounts for bulk purchases, or to book an event, please email dccpublishing@gmail.com or visit our website at: www.runandsmelltheroses.com.

Publisher's Note

Library of Congress Control Number: 2016943934

Library of Congress Cataloging-in-Publication Data
Run And Smell The Roses / Yolanda Diaz and Itarsha Payne p.cm

ISBN-10: 0-9912285-5-3
ISBN-13: 978-0-9912285-5-3

PRINTED IN THE UNITED STATES OF AMERICA
10 9 8 7 6 5 4 3 2 1

Dedicated to my daughter Megan. You bring me joy and pride.
You have always been a source of my inspiration.
Yolanda Diaz

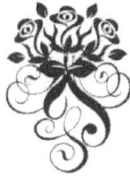

For you, Darryl Elijah. My first true heartbeat, my first true love, and the reason I never gave up. Love mom.
Itarsha Payne

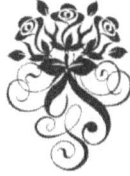

Contents

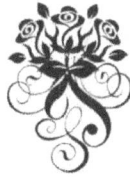

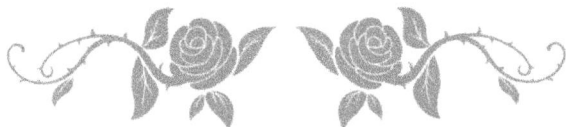

"SMELLING THE ROSES!"

Yes! We've said, "Smelling the Roses!" At times, as people, we all fail to stop and take a moment in life to just "Smell the Roses!" We often focus so much on the final destination or final outcome that we don't allow time to focus on the little things along the way; such as, life lessons, knowledge we can gain, or simply, the stuff right smack dead in our faces – the good stuff or not so good stuff!

For many of us, stopping to "Smell the Roses" is the same as that moment we stop, breathe, and say to ourselves, "I finally get it." It's that moment when things become **crystal clear**, that moment when things feel **just right**. It's a moment we can never duplicate, that one and only moment in time – that "AH-HA MOMENT."

Though those moments don't occur every day, when they do, we never forget them. Strange how we remember the date, time, and what we were doing when those moments hit. Some of those moments we cherish and learn from; however, there are some "Smelling the Roses" moments when we say to ourselves, "This is it, this is that pivotal moment, this is my turning point." That moment when we say, "I finally get it and I need to make a change and live it. I need to make that change NOW!"

As dedicated mothers and dedicated runners, we've documented our journey to becoming runners by sharing our journey and **ah-ha moments**, better known as our **Smelling the Roses** moments. We feel these important moments, as well as the great knowledge we've gained along the way, encompasses our achievements of becoming consistent runners, which we enjoy and continue to this very day.

Through running, we've learned so much about ourselves. During this journey, both of us have had many life changing experiences. We both have experienced physical setbacks and many twists and turns in our personal lives and careers, but through it all, we still continue to encourage one another and others. Through it all, we have been blessed to be able to continue to do what we love to do and that's RUN!

Throughout this wonderful journey we have become stronger, wiser, and happier with ourselves and with our lives.

God has given us this wonderful gift, the love of running, and because of this gift, we will continue to "Run and Smell the Roses!"

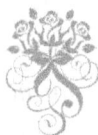

TIP

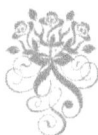

Make sure to take time to really enjoy your runs. Along the way and as often as you can, remember to **"Smell the Roses!"**

Yolanda

Well, I must say you never know when something is going to come your way and change your life, but as I get older and wiser, I am finding out life is always changing. I recall in 2004, as a 38-year-old single mother raising a teenage daughter, having any personal time for myself was mostly nonexistent. In 2004, any personal time that I had was dedicated to my daughter. My highest applause and respect to you single parents out there. During those days, I worked in the hotel industry, which never allowed me much personal time. I am one of those people who put a lot of time and passion into their career, especially one I enjoy doing. At the time, I was conscious of the fact that I would be turning 40 years old soon. I would always see magazines and television shows that would state when people get older; their metabolism slows down. At age 38, I really started to consider how I was going to keep my metabolism at least stable. Two years prior, my basic workout regimen was 30 minutes on the treadmill. When I turned 38, that exercise routine was not working as well as it did when I was 36. By the time I was the BIG 40, not only did my metabolism get slower, but my life changed. I, like many others, fell into the routine of forgetting about me. I did not continue to do any exercising for about three years. Within that three-year period, I continued my work in the hotel industry and during the latter part of those three years, I had become so knowledgeable of how to succeed in the hotel industry that I left the hotel industry. I became the proud owner of a large event facility. This facility helped people have wonderful and memorable events at an affordable price. I accomplished that mission and I will always feel proud of entrepreneurial experience.

In April of 2008, at the age of 41, my life changed again. After closing my business, I began to listen more to God and think about what was most important to me. I also stopped, reviewed, and evaluated the last three years of my life. I started to look at the age of forty-plus as a time to start a new beginning and to be the best example I could be from a fitness perspective, especially to be the best example for my daughter, Megan. Any parent can attest to the fact that when there is something that will help encourage and influence our children, then we will commit to doing it. In addition to influencing my daughter, I thought about how I wanted to be healthy when she became older and had children of her own. Based on these thoughts, my life was truly taking a new direction. It felt good to be thinking about me and getting to know ME for a change!

In 2008, I settled into a new job. This job involved less travel than my previous career in the hotel industry and allowed me to live a more organized life and schedule, as my daughter entered high school. This time in my life was a wonderful newfound feeling for me. I was now able to spend more time with Megan before she finished high school and headed off to college to start her career in nursing. Based on the direction my life was taking, I took the time to contact my friends that I had lost contact with over the years and Itarsha was one of them.

She is one of my dearest friends. Back in 1999, Itarsha and I worked in the same building. This particular building housed the hotel I was working for at the time and several other offices. Itarsha worked for an organization who had offices located in that building. It was so nice to see another tall woman wearing heels. We met one late afternoon at the front desk and have been friends ever since. We became instant best friends. We now know meeting each other was meant to be. I was in her wedding in 2002. Unfortunately, like I mentioned earlier, I had quit working out, so I was in her wedding—overweight, unhealthy, and unhappy. Work, work, work, and more work was my world back in those days. I truly love the hotel industry and being in sales. I was very driven to exceed sales goals. Years later, in 2008, I finally realized a life of all work and no taking care of "ME" is never good. I told myself, "You need and must have a good balance." When I realized that I needed a balance that is what I started to create for myself.

It was so great making the time to talk with friends again. After being reconnected with Itarsha in March of 2008, I mentioned to her that I was going on a cruise in September 2008. Also, I let Itarsha know that I had recently started walking in the early evenings after work to get in better shape for the cruise. Itarsha lived less than a mile from me. She said she would love to join me and walk with me. I was overjoyed and so excited about her joining me. We had told each other that we could use our walks to catch up on all the missed years.

Just from walking, I began to feel wonderful and experience my body making so many amazing changes. These were changes and feelings that I wanted to begin documenting. One morning, two years later, while Itarsha and I were walking, I made the suggestion to write a book and document our journey to fitness. Itarsha agreed, so we committed to each other to make it happen!

Itarsha, being back in my life, was God's doing for many reasons. As you can see, this fitness journey was one of them. Sometimes it truly does "take two to make a thing go right!" Two, meaning you and another, but also that two can be you and God; He is always with you. It is our hope that this book will inspire you and others to work together as a team to accomplish fitness goals or anything you want out of life.

Itarsha

I was always thin growing up. I had these long skinny legs and could eat anything I wanted and not gain a single pound! I even had a short bout with modeling as a teenager. Back then I never thought twice about what I put in my mouth. I couldn't gain weight even if I tried. However, all that came to a screeching halt after I had my son, Darryl Elijah. I was a single parent, until he was 11 years old, and though not necessarily proud of it, "eating-on-the-go" was sometimes our only option. With working full-time, raising Darryl and life in general, I began to put on weight and my body began to transition from thin to something I was just not happy with at all. I was never what one may call "fat" and wasn't considered overweight for my height. I'm 6 foot 1 inch and carried my weight all over my body versus in a concentrated area. When a woman is my height, she can carry weight better than someone not as tall, but 200 pounds is 200 pounds. Period.

My journey to the healthier lifestyle I live now began one day in January 2002. I went shopping for my wedding dress and the only wedding gown I absolutely loved in the entire bridal store didn't fit. Like I mentioned earlier, I wasn't considered overweight at 6 foot 1 inch and a size 14 (going into a 16), but on that day, it didn't matter; because the gown was a size 10. I wanted it badly, but couldn't pull it up past my hips. So what did I do? I bought the gown and I exercised and dieted to lose the weight. I comfortably slipped into my dream gown on my wedding day, nine months later. I never looked back and that was in September 2002.

I continued to exercise long after my wedding day and long after I reached my ideal bodyweight and size. I really enjoyed working out because I liked the way it made me feel. Throughout my journey, I've tried several different exercise programs and at-home-videos. Those awesome programs and videos are what got me into my wedding gown and down to my ideal bodyweight and size. However, the changes in my body, spirit, and mind that came from running cannot be compared to any other workout that I have ever experienced. That call from Yolanda back in April of 2008 changed my life. It had been over a year since I spoke to or even seen my very close and good friend Yolanda. I was elated when she called me to walk with her to get ready for a vacation she was going on that summer. Yolanda and I were no strangers to working out together. When I was on a quest to lose weight, Yolanda and I would workout at her house at times. We would use the treadmill, walk the neighborhood, or do home workout videos together. Yolanda was also in my wedding, (and there for me through my divorce), so see we have always been there for one another throughout the years. However, like it often can, life gets in the way sometimes, and though never far from your heart or thoughts, friends can become distant from your everyday life. That's what kind of happened. I settled into married life and Yolanda got married along the way and began running a new business. The first week we spoke, after that long hiatus, we agreed to start walking together. The weather was warming up. It was beginning to stay lighter longer and it was a healthy way for us to catch up on lost time. I know God put us back in each other's lives at the right time and that EXACT time by no mistake. Those short walks back in 2008 turned into five-mile runs three days a week. Unbeknownst to us, those walks would end up changing our lives.

It's said that everything happens for a reason and for a season. Yolanda returning into my life, at the very season that she did, was God's way of smiling down on me. At the time, I didn't know the reason, but now I know God knew there was no one else fit to walk this journey with me and I thank Him for it.

We both have a strong desire in our hearts and spirits to help others through memoirs of our journey of becoming runners. We want to see other women thrive and become all God designed them to be. We hope and pray with this documentation of our journey we are helping others, even if it is in some small way.

Chapter 1

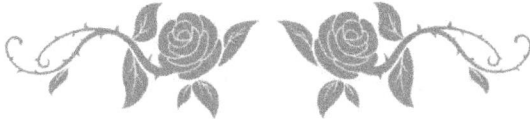

WHO WE WERE GROWING UP

Yolanda

I was born in Fort Bragg, North Carolina. My dad, Jamie Carlos Diaz-Kelly, is Panamanian, from Colón, Panama and a retired Army Master Sergeant. My mother, Delores Johnson, is African American and Native American Indian. She is from Fayetteville, North Carolina. I have a sister, Elvia Diaz that is one year younger than me. When I was about six years old, we moved from Fayetteville, North Carolina, because my dad got stationed at an Army base in Edgewood, Maryland. This is where I grew up most of my life and lived until the age of thirty. Fortunately for me, I was one of those kids that my parents shipped off since the age of seven every summer to stay with my grandmother in Fayetteville, North Carolina. While at my grandmother's house, a lot of times I would stay with my uncle, his wife, and two sons in Hope Mills, North Carolina. During those days, my uncle's wife's family had a farm with dirt roads. I loved going to the country each summer. I was, what some people call, a Maryland "Suburb Mouse" during the school year and a North Carolina "Country Mouse" in the summer. Growing up, I loved playing sports. My mother and father made sure my sister and I were involved in all kinds of activities. When my dad wasn't away on TDY (Army orders), he worked at his part-time job as a manager for the army base recreational center. While my father was working, my sister and I would be there all day, partaking in all types of activities, such as swimming, tennis, ping pong and many other activities. While living in army housing, I had the fortunate pleasure of living above a great family. A family with six kids that ranged from ages eight through sixteen — three boys and three girls. The older girls taught me dance moves and how to step. I was only ten years old and I was stepping like a college girl. I loved it! We would have awesome talent shows. The boys in their family showed me how to play marbles and catch frogs, as well as insects in the creeks. I can't believe I used to do that and loved it! This is an example of one family that lived in our building. In addition to that family, I also had the pleasure of growing up with kids in my neighborhood from Germany, Korea, Canada and from all over the world. Learning how to say German and Korean curse words was fun. As any army brat knows, when you have the pleasure of growing up with a parent in the military, you are exposed to many different cultures. I feel that was the beginning to the molding of my personality of being able to relate to all types of people so easily.

When I was eleven years old, my parents divorced. I was blessed with a strong, supportive mother who worked hard, while taking care of two children as a single mother and doing so, as my father continued to move to other locations as assigned by his Army career. My dad always made sure to keep in touch with us. God blessed me with great parents!

My mother is now and has always been a beautiful woman inside and out. She was the kind of mom that when she would come to school to see me, the guys would say, "That's your momma?" In my younger days, my mother was a model and helped to teach modeling for a school called Barbizon Modeling. In addition to modeling, she loved dancing and became a great tap dancer. My mother still enjoys all kinds of dancing and modeling today.

When my mom became an empty-nest parent with my sister and I living our lives, she continued to set her path on her passions. Living in Baltimore City, she became a community advocate for the NAACP. She owned an event facility in down-town Baltimore, near the Inner Harbor for many years. She also became the first minority awarded a contract as professional auctioneer for the City of Baltimore. After closing her event facility, she began her career in the medical industry. Currently in addition to her medical career, she still does auctioneering, volunteering and dancing.

My dad was and still is a very handsome man. While grow-ing up, he had slicked back soft hair and was known as the "other Ricky Ricardo." My dad did a tour in the Vietnam War in 1966 and 1967. He has always enjoyed sports. Boxing, basketball, football, and softball are a few of his favorites. He played on many softball teams while I was growing up and still plays even today! I guess that is why I love sports so much. Although my parents divorced, he was still a part of our lives, as much as he could be due to his Army career. He moved around a lot based upon his Army travel orders. He was in Germany, Texas, and Okinawa just to name a few—everywhere really. He still found time to help me purchase my first car, a Chevy Chevette. My dad remarried when I was 17 years old. After my dad retired from Fort Meade, Maryland, June 30,1991, he and my stepmom, Iris (a dedicated Science teacher) moved to Puerto Rico, where my stepmom is from. I am so proud of my Dad. After retiring, he obtained a degree in Microbiology. My parents' accomplishments in life have been an inspiration to me. My dad and my stepmom raised five children: Ivy Diaz-Lopez, Christina Diaz-Lopez, Gladys Diaz-Lopez, Iris Diaz-Lopez, and Jaime Jr. Diaz-Lopez. Including my sister, Elvia Diaz, I have a total of five sisters and one brother.

I was a very tall girl by 8th grade, 5'9 to be exact and by high school, 5'11. Yes of course, I was teased for my height. I was tall and thin. I was rightfully called Olive Oyl, the cartoon character, a lot. Being tall was bittersweet. As a senior in high school, those cruel boys would call me names like Larry Bird, the NBA player, and Big Bird from Sesame Street, but when I would go other places, people would ask me if I was a model or they would tell me you should be a model.

I was told so much that I should be a model that although I never thought of actually becoming a model, I was starting to consider modeling during my senior year of high school. I was a shy girl and afraid to go to a big city like New York. My perception of the modeling industry was at the time, one that I thought I would be alone in the Big City and exposed to the wrong things and people. So that perception kept me from pursuing modeling. I decided to pursue a career in Hotel Sales and Marketing within the hospitality industry.

In addition to my parents, my siblings are very talented and inspire me. My sister Elvia is working on her goal of becoming a nurse practitioner in addition to being an awesome cook and baker! Ivy has a degree in Criminal Justice and Microbiology, Christina has a degree in Microbiology, Gladys has a degree in Occupational Therapy, Jamie Jr., my only brother, is an accountant and a proud father of four, and my baby sister Iris, mother of an autistic son, has a degree in Occupational Therapy, as well.

As each member of my family is inspiring to me, I feel as the BIG SIS that I can help my siblings, family, and friends by being an inspiration for them as it relates to health. I hope that my quest to be healthier and fit will somehow, one day, motivate them and others to do the same in a way that works well for them.

~~~

Itarsha

At the very young age of 5 years old, my mother moved my older sister Johnna and I to San Bernardino, California. I was born in Brooklyn, New York, but we moved away shortly after my parents divorced. My mother and father, may they both rest in peace, were both African American and from New York. We lived in California for seven years and that is where my mom met my younger brother Jamel's father. At the age of twelve, we moved back to Brooklyn and that is where I lived, until moving to Raleigh, North Carolina in 1994 at the age of 22.

When I moved to North Carolina, my son Darryl Elijah was 2 years old, and I was on my own raising him as a single parent. There were a few reasons I moved from Brooklyn, New York; however, the main reason was I didn't want to raise my only son in the city. New York City, itself, also known as the Big Apple, is a great place to live depending on your circumstances. The theatre, performing and visual arts, and wonderful career opportunities are just a few reasons to live in New York. However, it is not the environment I felt comfortable with raising Darryl Elijah. I earned my paralegal degree straight out of high school. Shortly after receiving my degree, I landed a job with the New York public school system working as a paralegal for the Board of Education Hearing Office in Brooklyn. Boy did that job open my eyes to what I didn't want for my son! Darryl Elijah was only two years old at the time; however, I was thinking ahead, and I knew I would not feel at peace sending him to school after seeing firsthand what kind of negative activities took place in New York City high schools during that time. As a paralegal, at the Board of Education Hearing Office, I saw firsthand the criminal activities going on in the high schools. The cases crossed my desk, before being assigned to an attorney for a decision on the fate of the student who committed the infraction. Working there for almost two years was enough for me to make the decision to move south. I know I made the right choice. Darryl Elijah is now 25 years old, living his life as a responsible adult, praise God! His father has always, from day one, been in his life, though he lives in New York. So Darryl Elijah has always had all the love he needed from both of us.

As I mentioned previously, I was a tall, lanky girl growing up. By the age of 15, I was 6 feet tall and by the time I graduated high school, I was 6 foot 1 inch tall. I felt awkward from a really young age throughout my teen years due to my height. I have just always been tall. As a young girl, I struggled with my height. For a female, 6'1" is extremely tall and not common. I didn't go to sleep one night and wake up tall. I was always the tallest girl in the classroom. Heck, in junior high school, I remember being one of the tallest students in the entire school! In elementary school, I was often teased because I was much taller than the boys. Nothing changed in junior high or high school, so you can probably guess I didn't have a boyfriend throughout those years. Not having a boyfriend didn't bother me much because I was always too intimidated to talk to boys anyway. When I was young, I wouldn't speak to a boy first, even if it could have saved my life. Boys were intimidated by me, too. They wouldn't talk to me because of my height and I wouldn't talk to them because...well, they were boys! I was extremely shy and my tall stature made me self-conscious. Both personality traits don't go over too well at ages 12 through 17. To top things off, my mother had a tough time finding pants long enough and long sleeves were not even an option. So I could never wear the latest and greatest fashions. Due to the limited options for clothes, I had to wear anything that would fit my tall frame and I'm using the word "fit" loosely. Of course that left me with ill-fitting, unfashionable clothing. So to say the least, from 6th through 12th grade, I felt out of place in school, and around my friends. Period. Whenever my friends and I stood in a crowd, I would always stand behind everyone else in an attempt to hide my long body. I didn't want to stand out because I feared someone would make fun of my height or what I was wearing. When I think back to that time, I know I wasn't really hiding my tall frame, but I sure was trying my best not to stick out!

So I said all that to say: After dealing with the challenges of being tall over the years, unable to find clothes that fit properly, and getting way too much negative attention because of it, I didn't want to add size to the mix! As if being tall wasn't hard enough, after I had my son, everything I ate seemed to stick. My body just started to take on a different *shape* and *look*. Though I wasn't considered overweight for my height, I felt and looked "big" at the size I was, due (well you've kind of guessed it) to my height. I was very unhappy and self-conscious about the way I looked at that point more than ever before in my life.

A lot of women use shopping to help them feel better when they are feeling down. This act is known as "retail therapy." Well let me tell you, back then retail therapy was never "therapeutic" for me and as a matter-of-fact, shopping added insult to injury. Shopping was basically a nightmare! It was difficult to find clothes to fit right. Clothing designers don't typically design clothes for women over 5'6" to 5'8", unless the clothes come from a specialty store specifically for tall women. Well of course anything "specialized" also comes with a "special" price tag. I couldn't afford to shop at a specialty store. Besides, prior to being able to shop online, there weren't any stores accessible to me that sold tall women's clothing. So let me paint a picture of my shopping escapades back then. I would walk into a clothing store, pick up a blouse, and if it was a long sleeve blouse, I'd have to inspect the sleeves to see if it had cuffs or hems on the sleeves that could be let down, because I already knew the sleeves wouldn't be long enough. If by chance the cuffs could be adjusted, I'd also have to buy at least one size up for it to fit comfortable around the shoulders and torso. Nine times out of ten, the blouse would have to go back on the rack. Now, let's not even talk about pants or jeans! Buying pants off the rack was virtually impossible, so I wouldn't even try. They were all too short and again, I would have to go up in size, if I found a pair even remotely long enough to have the hem taken out. To top this off, I have scoliosis and my left leg is about ¾ to 1 inch shorter than my right. So, if I was lucky enough to find a pair of pants with a two-inch hem, then the left had to be let out more (if at all possible) to accommodate the right side.

Dresses and skirts were hardly ever long enough. If by chance I found an "okay" clothing item, it was nothing too cute. I couldn't shop for something to fit AND be cute, that was just too much to ask. I had to pretty much just shop for ANYTHING to just fit. So as you can see, none of this was enjoyable.

Let's fast forward to current day…I LOVE my height now, and the changes in my body that came with running has truly helped tremendously! I've come a long way! I can honestly say I love to shop, I love trying on clothes, and I love how I feel and look in my clothes; they just fall better on my body now than ever before. Guess what? I even wear 3 and 4 inch heels! It's definitely helped that I can shop online for clothes for tall women, unlike many years ago.

I've had parents of young girls or young girls themselves approach me to say how tall and beautiful I am, or how nice I look in my clothes, and to even admire that I have on heels. I have to admit; at first it was a bit uncomfortable to hear such compliments, because I wasn't mentally prepared to accept them. However, now I am. I always tell the parents of these young girls or the young girls themselves to hold their heads high because they are beautiful and unique. However, I know firsthand those words don't mean anything at all if they aren't carrying around the self-confidence within themselves.

I will never forget how my mother always, always said those exact words to me: "Stand tall with your shoulders back and NEVER slouch because you are unique, and you are beautiful." She told me that almost every day when I was growing up, but I never believed it, until now. I just thought those words were just things she was supposed to say because that's what mothers do.

I love my height now and wouldn't trade it for the world. It feels good to be different. Now I hold my head high with confidence. Did the transformation in my body give me the confidence I now have? Yes, indirectly it did. This journey truly played a huge role in getting me to the point of self-acceptance and realizing that I am unique in my own way. God made me this way and I now fully embrace my uniqueness. The mental transformation that came from running has allowed me to carry my confidence like a badge that I am proud of wearing.

Ladies, my ultimate goal for you is that you feel and truly believe how beautiful you are on the inside and out. There is only one you and no one can take your place in the world of your loved ones. Running helped me become a better version of me, and in my own little way, I hope I can help you get there, too!

Today, I live each day striving to be the best "ME" I know how to be. I do this by living a healthy lifestyle through the joy of running. I believe that life is too short, or too long, to be unhappy if you can help it. I hope sharing my journey of living a healthier lifestyle will help you in some way become the best version of YOU that you can be. Believe me, it's never too late!

Chapter 2

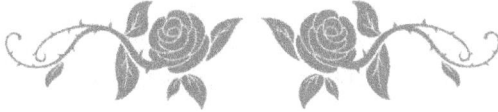

MAKING THE COMMITMENT

Making a commitment is the first step to change. Nothing is more important than you. If you don't take care of you, then YOU are unable to take care of others. Make the choice to change TODAY! Just by making the commitment then you are on your way to a better YOU.

In life, we often have a natural desire to map out in our heads what we want to commit to, and the possible outcome, before we actually make the commitment. Make no mistake, we understand the need and importance in mapping out certain roads of life and setting specific time-bound goals before embarking upon them. In some instances, it would probably be considered crazy or foolish not to plan. There are definitely times in our lives when mapping out specific goals first is essential, as it pertains to making a commitment.

A few examples of when a good thought-out plan and goal should be in place, before making a commitment, include getting married, going to college or back to college, building a home, and having children. However, there are times when it's not feasible to map out every detail to make a commitment.

Some journeys, such as ours, didn't come with a clear cut plan, exact destination, or specific directions. Every step was a new learning experience that led to another step, then another, and so on and so on. In the beginning, we basically "committed" to be committed to this journey, and then set goals. Through physical, mental, and spiritual growth, our journey became a very important part of who we are today and at the end of it all, that was the ultimate goal.

Our commitment began in **April 2008**. We began walking 30-40 minutes, Monday through Thursday in the evening after work. It felt so good to be doing this for ourselves. We alternated driving to one another's neighborhood. We continued this regiment throughout the summer of 2008. Then in **September 2008**, we changed our regimen to walking Monday, Wednesday, and Friday mornings at 6AM for 50-60 minutes. We continued this schedule of walking until **February 2009**. Up until this time, we hadn't logged the distance of our walks, but we had only logged the time. We always made sure we walked for no less than 50 minutes. The only reason we changed to morning walks versus night walks, is so we could have more time in the evening for family and running errands. That just worked for us.

In **February 2009**, we decided it was time to track our miles and distance, so we mapped out the route that we walked in each neighborhood. We set the car odometer to zero and drove each route to discover we were walking 3 miles within 50 minutes. Ironically, both our neighborhoods have several steep hills, but we did not let that discourage us.

After 9 months of consistent walking, our bodies built up endurance, and we had enough stamina to begin running. Your body will let you know when it's ready for the next level. By **mid-February 2009**, our morning started with running one mile and walking two miles. We began to run one full mile without stopping. This was a huge accomplishment for us. **By the end of March 2009**, we continued to run the first mile and also, built up enough stamina and courage to run 2 minutes and walk 5 minutes for 3 miles for a total of 4 miles. We had to go up several steep hills...OMG!!! However, at every level, our bodies and minds adjusted. This was a huge challenge for both of us. We were finally at a point where we wanted to add more distance with running. We set a goal to run 4 miles without stopping by **November 2009**. I know this sounds extreme, but we were really motivated and proud of our progress thus far. We felt we had met each goal set forth and 4 miles was within our reach. Only through consistency did our bodies began to get stronger and stronger from week to week. We noticed that we weren't as winded or tired after running. This allowed us to move faster toward reaching our goal.

In July 2009, we began to run 2 miles and walk 2 miles. We are proud to say that in **September 2009**, we met our goal of running 4 miles! September 2009 marked the month we official-ly became *"runners."* We began running a full 4 miles without stopping. We continued to run 4 miles three days a week for one year. **In September 2010**, we began running 5 miles three days a week. We joined a local gym to run on the treadmill on days when the weather was too cold, raining, or snowing. We did not have an actual goal to run 5 miles. Again it was only through CONSISTENCY that our bodies became empowered to push further. CONSISTENCY = ENDURANCE, STAMINA, DETERMINATION, and POWER.

We have only missed running together when one of us has gone on vacation or away on travel for work. We've run in 17-degree weather. This includes snow and some rain, when it wasn't outright pouring down. In hot or cold weather, we've run dark or light, we've run tired or not—we've run. Sometimes the inclement weather forces us to run on the treadmill, but we still get it done, no excuses!

We plan as much as possible around our running days, doc-tor appointments, work meetings, and anything else that might interfere with our run. We even refrain from taking any medica-tion that may cause drowsiness the night before our scheduled run. When we go on vacation or away for work, we verify that a treadmill is available in the hotel, so that we can run.

If we have to run 5AM opposed to 6AM so that one of us can make an appointment, then that's what we do! I can't pinpoint the moment or day that the dedication and determination kicked in, but it did early on and has been with us for many years. Is it easy? No, not at all, but the rewards far outweigh the sacrifices. We are proud of how far we have come and have no intentions of looking back. We know eventually the time may come when we want to do more than 5 or 6 miles a day. We know it's coming; however, we are very comfortable and proud of our dedication to the commitment we made. We could not have done this alone. The basis of our success is God First and our commitment to running as a team, second. Each day, one of us is waiting outside in our car for the other to walk out the door. We will not let each other down. We show up for each other every day.

We realized after two and a half years that the consistency caused us to make running a habit. We all know if we do something consistently, it will become a habit. Our minds and bodies have been transformed! We couldn't stop doing this even if we wanted to. After many years, running is part of our lifestyle and we want it to become part of yours, too. We want you to commit to running and run often. However, and more importantly, we want you to never outrun your joy of running.

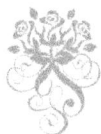

TIP

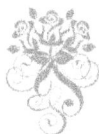

Running has given us the courage to start, the tenacity to keep at it, and the spirit to have fun along the way.

Itarsha "Smelling the Roses" on Making The Commitment

We are all committed to something, someone, or both. So most of us aren't strangers to being committed, and what it MEANS to truly be committed. With true commitment, comes sacrifices, expectations, give-and-take, time, patience, flexibility, understanding, and an open mind. Whew! When you break it all down, being committed seems like a fulltime job! So of course like any other commitment, it took time before I made the commitment to running and living a healthier lifestyle. So I guess it can go without saying, the commitment didn't come first, not by a long shot. I didn't just wake up one day and say to myself *I am going to become a runner*. I didn't watch an infomercial and decide I wanted to become a runner. Nor did I read or perform research on becoming a runner. My journey began slowly and was gradual. The whole thing just kind of snuck up on me.

Up until I made the commitment, working out was always the means to meet a short-term goal. For many years, I would occasionally workout before I made the decision to commit to this journey. I would often workout long enough to drop a few pounds and feel good about myself for an upcoming event or a vacation. Once the event or vacation came and went, I would stop working out. In an earlier chapter, I talked about how I worked out to lose weight to fit into my wedding gown. Even then, I had no plans to continue working out after my honeymoon. The commitment kicked in when I wanted to quit because there were so many other things like housework, shopping, etc. to do. I had to dig deep down inside and find the commitment to exercise on a continuous basis. I had to replace putting everything else under the sun first, with my love for running and it has been with me ever since. My commitment to running has truly changed my life in a way that I never thought possible. It's just not the physical changes; it's also the emotional gains that I've noticed. I think to myself on occasion that God gave me a gift—the determination and endurance to take advantage of the body he gave me. I am more focused and less stressed and in the best shape of my life!

I experimented with many different cardio workout regimens during my weight-loss journey. I did kickboxing, the elliptical machine, Pilates, and other exercise-related things, as well. I will never knock any of them, as they all played a role in helping me reach the point I'm at now.

Running has added so much to how I view fitness on a whole. I must say that I am grateful to have enjoyed the process it took to become a runner. Day after day, month after month, and even year after year, I still feel a sense of excitement before I embark on a run. When I tell people that I run 5 to 6 miles three times a week, some look at me like I'm crazy. *What is a "sista" doing running like that? What is she trying to accomplish? She is already thin.* Those are the comments I hear or that their eyes translate. Their remarks and behavior used to bother me, but I began to think to myself, God gave me these long legs and I made a commitment to myself, so I'm going to run!

Yolanda "Smelling the Roses" on Making The Commitment

To me, I feel in some instances this word "**COMMITMENT**" can be rather intimidating at times. Especially, when the word "**MUST**" is added to it, and even more intimidating, when you hear these words from someone else. When we started our journey to be fit, I decided I was not going to let those words intimidate me when it came to doing something for **ME**!

Committing to something for me and only me, gave me a whole new appreciation for the word! Wow, all these years I had committed to a job, my family, and friends, and yet, never thought about putting something that just involved me into a commitment. For example: I thought making sure the house was extra neat was more important. And, God forbid, if I had a large load of laundry looking at me, I would actually feel like I must get the laundry done first, before anything else. Don't get me wrong, I keep a clean house, but I was a little obsessive with mine.

Ladies, I finally figured it out, after many years, that I will work the laundry, house cleaning, and the cooking into my commitment for **ME...not the other way around.** YES, my family did adjust and adapted to my newfound commitment. When I contacted Itarsha, I had been walking by myself in the evenings after work for about a week. I cannot say that I could have or would have continued faithfully doing this alone, but when Itarsha said she would walk with me, my commitment was not only to myself, but to her as well. This way of thinking truly helped set the tone for the beginning of our journey to become fit and it continues to this very day!

After learning how to master staying committed to running, I realized that commitment to ANYTHING takes the same road. Whenever I find out that someone has accomplished something such as quitting smoking, getting a degree, mastering the art of a skill, or even being a stay-at-home mom etc., I am thoroughly proud of them, and they are all inspiring to me. Although this book is about running, we can all relate, because like me, one day they said, "Today I am going to make this commitment!"

From the very start, my commitment to running has brought me such wonderful rewards. It is so good to be able to say, "I did it." When you look back one month, three months, or even a year later, you will never ever forget the day that something totally different takes over you and said, "Today is the day!" Although I've never done illegal drugs, I can better understand the feeling of a drug addict that wants to quit. So often we've heard therapists say that nothing will happen until that person is **REALLY** ready to make a change. Don't ever let something keep you from the commitment you are ready to and want to make. Remember, it's a journey and journeys can be bittersweet. I can tell you that any journey to make yourself better is always less bitter and more sweet! AMEN! Your family and fans will be on this journey with you, and I've learned there will always be someone there to toot your horn.

Setting Your Goals

Ladies, stop now if you've set an UNREALISTIC goal of fitting into that size 6 dress in a week and you are a size 16. This is not the book for you. What this book is intended to do is to help you set realistic goals that are attainable once you make *the commitment* to become a runner. We are not saying that this will be easy because in our society we have been taught to expect and want instant gratification. We live in an "I want it now society." Both of us had to come to terms with the fact that there is no such thing as *health-in-a-bottle* and *fitness-to-go*. We quickly realized that we had to set realistic goals.

I know for us making the commitment, without setting goals right away, wasn't the hard part, because we knew it was time to DO SOMETHING! However, setting goals, when we didn't quite know what goals to set, was the difficult part. We knew we needed to reinforce our newfound commitment with ways to stay committed, which had to be goal setting. We had to set goals based on our lives and the world around us. The media over the past five to ten years consistently has drawn attention to health problems directly related to living an unhealthy lifestyle. Frequently, we would hear about a family member or friend who had health issues directly related to poor fitness. Based on this epidemic, we decided to now set goals to begin our journey.

So we first made the commitment to embark on our fitness journey. Once our commitment was firm and steadfast, we thought about what goals we wanted to set out to accomplish, while on our journey. We purposely broke our goals down into increments so that it wouldn't feel like such a huge undertaking. We began to focus on all the positive benefits that come from running and that became our motivation for setting goals. We have to say that the health benefits that can come from running are way high on our "goal setting" list. The positive health benefits within itself outweighed anything considered negative about running such as early mornings, social sacrifices, etc. by a long shot. Each goal set in essence was part of the plan to reach our bigger ultimate goal, and that was to become physically, mentally, and emotionally healthier and fit.

Make a list of all the positive benefits you can think of that can come from running and anything you deem as negative benefits that can come from running, and we can almost guarantee you that it will be easy to set your goals just by looking at your list. As you can see, we had to revisit our goals from time to time to remain on track, and you will need to do the same. As each goal set forth is met, a new goal should take its place. Fitness is like knowledge; you can never be too fit or healthy.

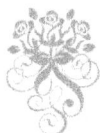

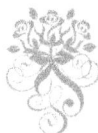

TIP
You are not running
for future rewards...the rewards start now!

Yolanda "Smelling the Roses" on Setting Your Goals

As I reflect on the word *GOALS*, I wonder why I would only set goals for my job and never set personal goals for me. Although it's very satisfying and motivating to have a job with performance goals, the goals mainly benefit the company. Now I think differently, and not only set goals for my career, but for my personal growth as well.

I remember playing sports in high school. All the things we learn when playing sports are lifetime lessons of reaching goals to win. It is no different with you as an individual, two, or only a few people. If you want to succeed at **ANYTHING**, a goal must be set. I always found it quite fun to self-challenge myself when I played sports in high school and field hockey in college. I would set a goal and a vision to score a certain amount of points. During my career advancement in the hospitality industry, I would set sales and marketing goals for myself far above what my employer wanted because I wanted to always exceed expectations and that brought me and my employer many rewards. I ask myself now, as we document our fitness journey, why I did not practice this concept of setting more personal and fitness goals? Let me tell you, I know now (I wish I knew this a long time ago) that there is NOTHING more satisfying than setting and reaching a goal that benefits YOU! When I set my goal to begin this fitness journey with something as simple as an evening walk, it made me feel so good! Especially, when I realized, I established consistency in doing something just for me. I find myself often thinking about if I would have started this journey and setting goals at age 25 or younger, how far along I would have been. However, it started when I was 41, and that is okay. It's okay if your age is 50, 60, or 70. Set your goals for you, today, and make them happen. Don't let anything keep you from them. You will see the results and realize that it was all worth the effort. I can testify to you on that and will provide any help that I can for you, too! You deserve it!

Itarsha "Smelling the Roses" on Setting Your Goals

I used to have a goal to run marathons and run longer distances. These were goals that I set when I first became a runner. At the beginning of my journey, I used to think that's what running was all about. I was supposed to run in races, challenge others, and challenge myself. I thought I was supposed to want to cut time off my runs, run faster, run harder, and always beat the time of my last run. However, that has since changed. Honestly, those feelings of reaching those goals and truly wanting those things never really kicked in at all. My main goal now, and even early on, when it comes to running, is to simply not quit.

One thing that stands true about goals is that they can often change, as we gain experience and go through life. I think the ability to be flexible enough to reposition myself and reset my goals based on unexpected occurrences has helped me stay on track with running. What I had to really get in my head and be mindful of is that "life happens" while I'm "making plans" to do things my way. In the beginning, I would get frustrated if I got off track due to being a little under the weather and not being able to run. Sometimes, I would get frustrated returning from vacation and not getting in all my miles for the week. I had to learn that flexibility is vital to reaching a goal because life happens no matter what plans I make. Once I accepted that it's okay to miss a run or two, and still stay on track with my over-all goals, my runs became even more enjoyable. Running slowly went from being just exercise to one of my passions. I no longer put undue pressure on myself when something beyond my control puts me a little off track. I've learned to just roll with the punches and know that as long as I've not lost sight of my overall goal as a runner, then I'm still on track even with a few missed runs. My journey is ongoing with no time frame. I want to be able to run as long as I enjoy it, and hopefully, that is a very long time. I know that you are probably thinking, *"What's the point of a goal, if it doesn't include a time frame? Isn't that what goals are all about?"* I have to say that you are absolutely right. Goals should be reachable and time-bound and some of mine still are. However, somewhere along the way I stopped putting a time frame on those particular goals. What I think would happen is that it would be counter-productive for me. If I were to put that kind of pressure on myself, what I appreciate and love about running would then become this horrible chore that I despise having to do. So my main and most important goal, when it comes to running, is to never lose my commitment and determination. With this first and foremost, I will continue to do what I love and that is to continue to simply run.

Am I telling you to not set time-bound goals? Not at all. Yes, there is nothing wrong with setting reachable time-bound goals.

Just remember the most important thing is to not get too focused on setting goals and putting yourself on a tight schedule to meet those goals. In so doing, it can make you miss out on appreciating the progress that you have made during your journey towards those goals.

Remember that setting goals should be looked at as motivation to strengthen your dedication and commitment, but don't put too much pressure on yourself. What's most important is that you have fun and enjoy the gift of running.

Defeating Excuses

Sometimes it is so hard to put YOU first. When we started this journey, in the beginning, it was hard to roll out of bed at 5:30 am and be out the door by 5:45 am. How did we do it? We did it by not listening to excuses that used to pop up in our minds:

- *It's too early.*
- *It's too cold.*
- *I just got my hair done.*
- *I went to bed too late.*
- *I'm still sleepy.*
- *It's okay to miss a run.*
- *I have a long day ahead.*
- *I deserve a "day off".*
    Etc., Etc., Etc....

The list goes on and on. So in the beginning to help us NOT come up with excuses, we made a pact. Our agreement is to not call in the morning and check-in to see if the other is running because it's set in stone…we are running! The idea to not call and confirm our scheduled runs makes it easier to not come up with excuses. So all we know, when we wake up is, "My friend is up and waiting for me to get there to start our run." That is what keeps us going. Knowing we need each other, there is NO EXCUSE for letting the other down. This approach works for us like a charm!

Once you learn to tune out the excuses in your mind, come up with a plan for them, fight them, push them aside, overcome them, and ultimately conquer them, so that it will become second nature to you like it has for us. This will help to get your run in with no excuses. Sooner than you think, you will begin looking for ways to always get your runs in and not ways to get out of running.

To our surprise, there were times when we had to deal with friends and family giving us what they deemed as excuses for us to not run. Believe it or not, and as strange as it may sound, there will be times when you will hear excuses for you not to run from your friends, family, and co-workers, etc. More than likely, friends and loved ones mean well and have good intentions (Hopefully, when they handout "their" perceived excuses about "your" fitness journey). What they fail to realize is that their advice can at times come off as negative and unsupportive. Unfortunately, this unsolicited advice better known as "excuses" is enough to rain on your parade…

- *You are going to ruin your knees!*
- *You shouldn't do this! You shouldn't do that!*
- *You're Crazy!*
- *You are losing too much weight!*
- *You don't need to run THAT much!*
  Etc., Etc., Etc.…

So with that being said, we have naturally learned to lean on each other for support. No one knows better, or cares more about your commitment or journey than the one that runs by your side and has the same goals in mind and that comes by leaning on each other. So you see in the beginning of our journey, once we pushed through our own excuses not to run, we had to contend with our families and friends giving us advice, excuses, and reasons why they thought we shouldn't run. Though we politely listened to their reasons, and smiled and nodded while hearing their advice, we continued to stand steadfast with our goals in mind. Fortunately, they finally realized that offering their excuses was a waste of their time because we were truly committed.

Once they realized that we were serious and dedicated, not only did they begin giving us accolades, they begin telling us how great we looked and actually began wanting to know what to do to possibly begin their own fitness journey!

Excuses: Hair, Weather, Tired, Appointments, Wanting to Socialize

Hair

Do not let your hair be an excuse. We both know firsthand how much of a challenge ethnic hair can be when it comes to working out. Find a hairstyle that will work for your running days. Weave, wigs, natural, buns, lace fronts, braids...there are a lot of great options for your hair to stay healthy and looking good.

Weather

We are always as prepared as we can be. If we think it will rain, we already have a Plan B in effect, which is going to the gym and running on the treadmill. We know the treadmill isn't always desirable, but it will keep you on track and that's important when the weather is not conducive to running. Do not let the weather keep you from your goal.

Tired

Being too tired could be an excuse for us every single day, but we will not let it be an excuse. We just get up! We don't fret or negotiate with our minds. We rise out of bed and get right to running. We are up, dressed and out within 15-20 minutes. Just think, you have to get up anyway, so what's an hour earlier?

Appointments

Running is an appointment, so we don't let other appointments keep us from running. If we can, we try to schedule any appointments around our running schedule. If that's not possible, we will run early if necessary. No matter what, we still find the time to run and it feels great to not let anything or anyone keep us from running.

Friends

As we mentioned earlier, your friends can create excuses and reasons for YOU not to run. Not just health related reasons and excuses, but way more enticing and immediate sacrifices. If you decide to run in the evening or after work, your friends can find better or more amazing things for you to do. The mall, a movie and popcorn, or a nice meal at your favorite restaurant will always sound better than running even to the most fit and disciplined individual. Though we run in the morning and don't have this particular issue, it can be one for you evening runners.

Our overall point when it comes to excuses: Ladies, anything worth having doesn't come without hard work and some sacrifice. Your fitness and health, inside and out, are priceless investments that can't be bought except through hard work, sacrifice, and overcoming excuses.

Itarsha "Smelling the Roses" on Defeating Excuses

Okay. I think I might hurt someone's feelings on this one, but STOP IT! Stop giving all of those excuses as to why you can't run, workout, or even move in some way! Unless you have physical limitations or a medical reason for not moving your body, NO EXCUSE is a good enough one.

I know, I know, you are giving me the stink eye for saying what I just said. However, ladies, I can talk because I have been there. I used to come up with all kinds of reasons to not workout when I know I needed to workout. What's sadder is that once I came up with the excuse, and convinced myself it was valid, I was completely satisfied with it. Well that was up until the day I was standing in a dressing room in a wedding gown that wouldn't zip. That's the very day I was fresh out of excuses.

Let me see if I can remember some of my favorites: "I'll start Monday. Yes, Monday is perfect for a fresh start." Of course, Monday never came. Another one I would use is: "I'm tired from running around all day at work and besides, that's considered exercise anyway." Oh and here is the best of the worst types of excuses, "No one else I know is exercising and they all seem happy, so what's the point?" That's a horrible excuse! Some of the other excuses I used were, "I'm tired," "I'm in school," "I have to cook, clean, and take care of my family," "I have errands to run," etc. etc. We all have the same challenges. Yolanda and I have experienced everything I stated above, but it doesn't stop us. I used to work full-time as a property manager, which means my work was never done, and I was on call 24 hours a day. When I started this journey, I was a wife, mother and a student. However, I know if I'm not happy with me, I wouldn't have the ability to make others around me happy. I can't give or spread what I don't have. I can't stress enough how important it is to take care of "YOU."

Okay ladies, my African American sisters, we all know our number one (numero uno) excuse on the list of excuses is our hair! Trust me, I feel your pain, and I know your plight, but at the end of the day a hairstyle is not worth it. I struggled (and still do at times!) to do something with my hair. I've had weave, ponytails, wigs, lace fronts, braids, and so on and so forth. Keeping my hairstyle is truly a challenge. However, trying to wear the latest hairstyle is not worth my health. It's just not that serious, and I want for you to feel the same when it comes to living a healthy lifestyle. I don't want to hear any excuses. Please ditch the latest and greatest hairstyle and put your health first! Stop the excuses today! Make your list of positive and negative reasons for running or fitting any workout regimen into your schedule...I know which list will win!

Ladies, we all can find a reason not to do something since it's just easier. I'm here to be your cheerleader, your coach, and your friend. I promise you, if you can push past the excuses, then you will be so proud of yourself!

Yolanda " Smelling the Roses" on Defeating Excuses

I am going to keep it really real with you. I have come home many days from a long day at work, eaten dinner, and felt there is no way I am running tomorrow morning. I am mentally and physically exhausted. Now keep in mind, I am saying this as I am laying out my running clothing gear for the next day (my brain is trained to do this). Then I start to think it's going to be 28 degrees tomorrow. At this point, I have stressed myself out about running the next day and now, I am eating out of a tub of ice cream and searching for chips frantically… LOL (I'm working on stopping that)! I told you I was going to keep it real. I finally get in bed and think about my overall day and realize, I can't let the stress of day to day life make me change my attitude towards my running commitment to me. Before falling asleep, I would say to myself, "Well, I guess I gotta run now, since I ate ice cream and ½ a bag of chips." LOL!

Honestly, the next morning I am recharged and immensely motivated. When I wake up, my brain is on schedule and is telling me, "Come on, let's go. I can't wait to get out there and run." Now let me remind you, I said my "brain" not my "body." My body jumps on board with my brain after the first ten minutes of running. That is what happens when you do something consistently. You are training your brain.

As I mentioned above, "my brain is trained to do this." I trained it to think this way. God gives us a tool to do what we need to and it starts in your mind. A baby can go from crawling to walking. We have all witnessed the journey of a crawling baby and their journey to their first step. We all are born with something in us to do what we need or want to do.

I finally learned to not spend my evenings, after work, worrying about my next morning run, the weather, or anything negative. I began to enjoy my life in each moment and you should, too. I have adopted the attitude that nothing can keep me from taking care of me or keep me from supporting our commitment to this journey. Missing a run is impossible, if we can help it. There will always be a million excuses, but you have to train your brain to focus on your goal and not allow anything beyond your control to allow you to make excuses.

For example, when Itarsha is out of town, which leaves me by myself to run, I could make excuses. Here are the excuses that come to my mind. I shouldn't run because, one, I need the rest; two, I should not go alone; three, I'll skip today and make it up another day. As soon as I stopped allowing the excuses for not running to enter my brain, I immediately started to allow thoughts of the reasons why I *should* run to enter. The truth is: Once you begin and you see the benefits, you will not make excuses.

Now, here are the solutions to the excuses I would create:

1. I need the rest;

    Solution:
    I can go to bed earlier tonight, if I need more rest.

2. I should not run alone.

    Solution:
    I can run when it's light outside, run the route that keeps me close to activity on the street, take my pepper spray, and a pouch around my waist to accommodate additional items of protection.

3. I'll skip today and make it up another day.

Solution:

Ha! Ha! Ha! I know realistically this would most likely not happen, and it would mess up my entire weekly running cycle. I want my regularly planned Saturday off as much as possible, so I definitely ditched this excuse.

Despite all the excuses I can use, I choose to get up and get going. It's YOUR motivation and YOURS ONLY that is going to keep you from making excuses. At times, you are going to have to do this alone. Stay true to you and your goal.

Chapter 3

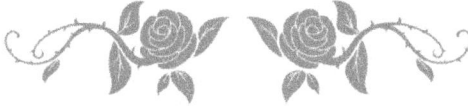

HEALTH STATISTIC

We know for African American and Hispanic women, basically all women of color, your curves are important to you, and we are not exempt! We love the curves the good Lord gave us! We are just as proud as you are to be blessed with curvatious hips and thighs. God made us this way, and as women of color, we should and will continue to embrace them.

In our culture, curves are considered to be a beautiful attribute and sexy on a woman. We believe that will always be the case and some of us even go as far as to "buy" curves to achieve a sexier look. It's become very popular over the years to enhance butt and hips with injections and/or surgery. Doing so is a very personal choice, and every woman has the choice to do what they want with their bodies. With that being said, we have to mention the not so good part of having too many curves, or curves in all the wrong places to where you're considered overweight or obese.

Research has shown us that obesity in the African American community and with women of color is on the rise. Based on research as well as observation, 4 out of 5 African American women are overweight or obese and 3 out of 4 Hispanic women are overweight or obese as well. Research has also shown that people who are overweight are more likely to suffer from high blood pressure, diabetes, high cholesterol, and are at risk for heart disease. It's also been stated that deaths from heart disease are almost twice the rate for African American women as compared to other nationalities. What's more alarming is that obesity in our children and teens are at a rise at almost the same rate as adults. Parents, we need to be good examples for our children because they look up to us, and we are their first role models.

We are in no way putting ourselves out here to be professionals when it comes to nutrition, exercise, and diet. However, we have done our fair amount of research and these are concerning findings that we want to bring to your attention. You can research more statistics by talking with your doctor, a nutritionist, or going on the Internet.

This knowledge we've gained from research and trial and error has really driven us to write this book. We want to not only change our lives for the better; we also want to help you change yours. Together, we can change the lives of our children. Let's start now, today!

Itarsha "Smelling the Roses" on Health Statistics

Sound the alarm!! I can't tell a lie. It doesn't look good for us. As we just mentioned, according to statistics, 4 out of 5 of us are overweight or obese! That means out of 100 women in church, a restaurant, a movie theatre, a concert, a stadium, or any kind of public event or venue, only 20 of those women, which includes strangers, co-workers, friends, and family are considered of a healthy size and weight.

Ladies, we have got to do something about this, but if not for ourselves then for our children! We can't ignore this and pretend like it will just get better on its own. As time goes on and we become more and more of a society of "we want it now," many things around us are being made easier to access and that includes food. On just about every corner and up and down every nonresidential street, there is a fast food or takeout restaurant. In most instances, we don't even need to get out of the car. We can just call in the order, pull up to the restaurant and voila, we have a yummy plate of food in front of us in way less time than it takes to take something out of the refrigerator to cook. Furthermore, some of the schools have fast food available for lunch brought in by a variety of fast food restaurants. I guess this is to give our children the freedom of "choice." The best thing we can do for ourselves and our children is to take this matter into our own hands. Before we can tackle these issues and concerns head-on, you need to fully understand what's working against you, and how your thinking, actions, and attitude can be the very thing holding you back from making those healthy changes you have wanted to make in your life.

Look around, we are right in the middle of the fitness-rage of the century! Almost everywhere you turn, somebody is talking about wanting to get fit or drop a few pounds. However, we have a few issues we need to overcome. First thing is, wanting a quick fix. Pretty much, like everything else in life, and as I mentioned earlier, we want it quick and we want it now! What I have noticed is that more of the people that I know, including people on television and social media, talk about living healthier lifestyles. However, many of these individuals only "talk" about wanting to get fit and don't really do or seek out what they need to do to actually work towards being fit, or becoming fit as a real, true lifestyle change. I think some people look at fitness as some kind of "fad" or something "cool" to do. Some individuals think short-term. They'll workout and eat healthy to fit into an outfit for a special occasion or to look good for an upcoming vacation. However, after that time passes, they go right back to their old habits. How do I know this you ask? Well that's because I used to do it a lot. My body knew the drill. Right after planning a trip or jotting down that date on the calendar for a party or special occasion, I went full throttle into diet and exercise. I would say to myself, "Okay, on Monday I'm not playing anymore games. I'm going to exercise and eat right." Monday would come and I would completely focus on losing weight JUST to look good for my trip or outfit for my upcoming event. Then as soon as the time comes and goes, I'm back to only wishing I could drop a few pounds and back to doing nothing about it. The cycle would start again as soon as another vacation or special event was booked. Whew, what a vicious cycle!

Second thing, the money makers and companies looking to make a profit capitalize over our determination to have everything quickly accessible with very little effort as possible. Everywhere you turn, there are new gadgets that claim you can do something or another for five minutes a day and look like the spokeswoman or spokesman modeling their product. Ladies, don't fall for the propaganda. I did many years ago and learned, it will not work, unless you WORK IT! I am here to tell you and help you. It takes hard work, time and discipline. I know you have it there inside of you, and I am here to help you find it, pull it out, and work it!

Though I feel strongly and feel that you need to be disciplined and do the work for positive long-term fitness changes, I have to come to the defense of African American and ethnic women everywhere. Growing up, we pretty much ate what our mommas put in front of us and at times, it wasn't considered the healthiest of choices. Our parents many times chose hearty over healthy (with love of course). It was important that we didn't go to school, go outside to play, or go to bed hungry. Ethnic food is often rich in fats for flavor and heartiness and many times ethnic food was whatever our parents could afford to put on the dinner or breakfast table, so as to fill us up.

I've personally noticed that most times the cheaper the food is, the less healthy it may be for the body. For example, fresh fruits and vegetables are sometimes more expensive, than canned goods, or an item off the "value menu" at some fast food restaurant. A couple of "value menu" items off a fast food menu will probably fill you up more than a banana or apple that may cost the same amount. So it's difficult to break a cycle of something we know so well. Also financially, many of us need to get "more bang" for our buck, so even though the meal may not be healthier to eat, it's more economical to eat. Eating healthy to take care of our bodies is just something that our community doesn't work hard to make a priority because our frame of reference in doing so may be null to none.

There is absolutely nothing wrong with our beautiful curves. I love what curves I have, and I know you love your curves as well. We should! Furthermore, our African American and ethnic men love and adore them, too! However, we really have to get off the surface and look so much deeper than that. Living a healthier lifestyle has never been more important than it is now, especially as we grow older and possibly face other health risks.

There are some things in life that are just unavoidable, even when it comes to our overall health, and there isn't much we can do to change some of these things. However, taking control over living a healthier lifestyle is something we have complete control over. It takes a little work, dedication, and commitment, but it's all worth it in the end!

Yolanda "Smelling the Roses" on Health Statistics

As a Hispanic and African American woman, these statistics sometimes feel like a double whammy to me. Do you hear what I hear? Are you in tune with what the recent health statistics are saying? Do you see what I see? Have you seen the size of children and teenagers lately? Do you notice that in a room with twenty women, chances are there is only 2%-5% that are within a healthy weight range and because of that, I have got to take control of this situation and say, "NO, this will not be me."

Well, a few years ago, I decided to take everything in perspective and decided that I wanted to be the one in the room of twenty women, who is within the healthy weight range.

Prior to running, I sat at a desk on a computer 80% of the time. I would often think if I don't do some type of exercise I could become very unhealthy. When you have a job where you sit all the time, like I had, with no form of exercise, you leave yourself vulnerable. I made a choice to be the minority instead of the majority, to help myself and others. Every now and then, some statistics can make you feel like you should be molded into looking a certain way. Well a statistic is basic information that you use to your advantage. You do not have to be a size two to be healthy, so never let any media information make you feel that you are not beautiful or healthy. The key is to use the information to be or become the best version of a beautiful and healthy you that you can be. Healthy is a feeling, not a size! You will know exactly what I am talking about as you begin your journey.

Consult With Your Physician

In many chapters, we have recommended that you speak with your physician, or to perform research on the Internet about that particular topic. The reason we consistently reiterate this throughout many of the chapters is because it is very important to get their professional advice, as we are not professionals. Remember ladies, we are speaking based on personal experience as well as trial and error. Consulting a physician should always be first and foremost.

By consulting with your physician, your physician can give you personalized and customized information, as well as the best perspective, based on your individual circumstance. Doing so will also allow your physician to suggest other resources, or additional testing you may need before starting such a regimen as well as any exercise routine. It may also be a great idea to consult with your physician when embarking upon changing your eating habits or diet. Your doctor may even suggest you see a cardiologist or specialist, based on your individual fitness level to maximize your overall fitness journey.

Your physician can give you great tips on the best running style for your body type. Whatever they suggest you to do, or don't do, please follow their advice over ours, at all times. They know **YOU** best.

Take a list of questions you may have about what you want to accomplish and inform them that you are beginning to embark on being healthier and fitter by running. I'm sure they will be proud of you and be more than happy to help you reach your fitness goals. Ladies, your doctors are a wonderful resource, so use them and listen to them.

Itarsha "Smelling the Roses" on Consult With Your Physician

Keeping my physician abreast of my physical activity is very important because of my health history. I was born with a mild to medium case of scoliosis, and I didn't know whether running would be beneficial or cause a negative impact further down the line. I didn't want to end up doing more damage to my spine, so his advice and feedback has been extremely vital to me. My doctor is equally a family physician and sports medicine physician, so he is well versed in the mechanics of the body and physical activity. I feel blessed to have such a physician on my side!

I've been seeing my doctor for a very long time. He knows my medical history inside and out. When I became really serious about running and moving toward a healthier lifestyle, he was one of my biggest supporters. Prior to that, he expressed his concerns about me getting older and how my scoliosis could progress. He never pushed me to begin a regular workout routine, but he always wanted me to be aware that with his experience with scoliosis, he's seen the condition progress negatively the older his patients were and the less active they became. Thankfully my doctor not only encouraged, but also assured me that it's completely safe to run as long as I'm not experiencing any mild to severe discomfort. One thing he did do, and I'm thoroughly grateful for, was equipped me with tips on how to get the best out of my runs, as well as gave me the dos and don'ts as it pertains to my scoliosis. Want to know what's amazing? I have less lower-back pain when I remain active. I still feel a mild level of pain pretty much daily, but it's not as prominent as it used to be before running. Actually, my back feels better now than ten years ago. Every time I see my doctor, he notices small improvements in my posture, and it's all contributed to running. For me, this is a huge deal because I've always, and to this day, still have a negative awareness and consciousness about my curved spine. So to not only hear that the scoliosis is not getting worse, but to hear there are small improvements is another blessing to me.

The last time I was in my doctor's office, he couldn't believe how great my posture had become. He beamed with pride and basically told me to keep doing what I'm doing and that I'm in the best shape he's ever seen me in so far. That felt really good to hear and was a good dose of encouragement.

Don't underestimate the advice of your physician. Let your physician help you get on the right track to living a healthier lifestyle. He or she may be able to shed light and elaborate on ailments and health complications directly related to carrying around excess weight and help you set goals to be that healthier version of you. I encourage you to use all of your resources. You are so worth it!

Yolanda "Smelling the Roses" on Consult With Your Physician

When I first began running, I reached out to my physician, and she was very happy I did. My physician is quite fit herself. She gave me some great tips and referred me to speak with a couple of orthopedics that could provide more of the dos and don'ts of running. You will have to take all the advice that is given and make your best judgment. Having some guidance is always good and appreciated. And, it has all helped me and continues to do so to this day. A short time after I began running, I decided to take things a step further by going to see a cardiologist. I had been told in my teenage years I had a slight heart murmur. When I went for the appointment I was a little nervous. My heart was hooked up to all these wires. It can put you in panic mode as you watch the doctor looking at monitors and saying nothing! When he finished, he asked me to wait for him in the next office over.

When he finally came in to go over the results he said, "Well, I have got some bad news for you." I replied with a deep breath, "Okay, I can handle it." He proceeded to say, "Well, my dear, you are going to have to keep on doing what you are doing because your heart looks fantastic!" He applauded me for listening to my inner spirit of taking things a step further to see a cardiologist. That experience helped me realize that a plane or a car does not take off until it goes through all the checks and balances. We must treat are bodies the same way. I could have use the fact that I had a slight heart murmur as an excuse and never started running. Listening to my inner spirit put me on a better road.

Find yourself a physician that you like and one that is an advocate for your journey. Spend a little extra on that copay to see a specialist for your feet, knees, back, and legs. Get to know your physician/s and ask them about their fitness routine. Get some extra information from those doctors in exchange for the extra money you're spending on that co-pay. Once your doctors are aware of your journey, they will become one of your advisors and they will become one of your fans.

Start Small

Honestly, we NEVER thought in our wildest dreams that we would become runners. Who, us? Two ethnic women that have full-time careers, family obligations, and at the time, over the age of 35. No, we didn't quite fit the bill. However, here we are many years later, dedicated to running and helping others follow in our footsteps. We are not only speaking to our ethnic sisters, we are also speaking to women of all backgrounds and all ages. It's never too late because the key is to just start small.

We believe to make any type of change in your life you should start small. Especially, if you desire it to be a long lasting and long-term change. We both completely understand that sometimes life forces us to take the bull by the horn and go full throttle. Those times are most likely when our back is up against the wall, and the only way to get results is to go fast and to go hard. However, this isn't an approach that any one wants to take 100% of the time. Handling change in this way all the time can be extremely exhausting and can be counterproductive depending on what the change is that one is facing. Furthermore, handling change in that way, can be tiring and stressful. This approach can also cause us to drop the ball or burnout if we are trying to do too much too fast. So starting small is essential in most cases if for no other reason than to keep us sane and safe!

Beginning a running regimen is definitely no different. Remember this is a lifestyle change. So fitting this change into your routine may require some adjustments and sacrifices before you find a consistent schedule that works for you. By starting small, you can easily begin to adjust to "the commitment" you made so that it will not dramatically disrupt your day-to-day routine. Starting small will also give your family and friends the opportunity to get used to the adjustments that you will need to make in your life that may indirectly affect them. At first, it may seem impossible to fit running into your schedule, but will soon be something that you look forward to and will become second nature to you.

We can all agree that it comes very easy to make excuses to avoid doing anything physical, especially early morning or after a long day at work or school. So any old reason or excuse to not go running will do. So the first thing is to start small by not putting running in place of any other obligation you have in your life. You will find that as you become closer to reaching your goal to becoming a runner, you will automatically make it one of your top priorities.

Starting out, you need to just fit running in where you have the existing "time" to do it. In the evenings, instead of watching T.V. or talking on the phone, go out for a walk or a run, or hit the treadmill at the gym, or the treadmill collecting dust at your house. If you are a morning person, wake up just 30 minutes earlier in the beginning and walk or run for 30 minutes before you shower for work. We all have a time throughout the course of our day that we can spare. It's what we decide to do with that spare time.

In the beginning, we found that the more and more we filled our spare time with walking and/or running, the more we MADE time for it. After a while, we no longer just filled our spare time with running, but we designated a time for our running. Which meant, we actually began to make running a priority and not just something to do in our spare time. However, this took time. It didn't happen overnight. Starting small was the glue that made it stick.

So how did starting small get us to where we are today with our commitment to running? Well, when we wanted to work walking and/or running on to our priority list, we did so by setting that as a goal. That was actually the goal, to simply make running one of our many priorities. It was as simple as that. When we felt the time had come and when it felt right, we both determined that we wanted to do more than to just fit walking and/or running into our spare time. So together we came up with ideas on how to do that, and we met that goal. That's it! One "small" goal and figuring out how to transition our running from a "spare time" activity to a "priority activity" was it. Doing it that way, kept us from overwhelming ourselves.

It's important not to think too far in the future when starting small as it will only overwhelm you. You are not in a race with anyone, so remember starting small will give you the tenacity and focus to stick with and live out your goal of becoming a runner.

After meeting our goal of shifting walking and/or running from a spare time activity to a priority activity, we made another small goal to begin walking 30-40 minutes four days a week. This was something else small and easily attainable for both of us. We first started walking in the evenings. We did this for a little while, and it was working out fine for both of us. After about two months of walking in the evenings, we both agreed that mornings were much better for our schedules. The sacrifice to change our walk-schedule and GET UP at 5am to walk was an adjustment, but a new priority, so we just did it. We made the adjustment to run in the morning for various reasons:

1. It fit our lifestyle and day-to-day routines.
2. We had more energy in the morning.
3. We had more time in the evenings for family and friends.
4. Our jobs, at times, required us to work late.
5. Last but not least, evenings cut into our mall shopping time!

Are we saying that by starting small, you will never feel discouraged or fall short? Absolutely not! There are many days, even after many years of running, when we think to ourselves: "This will be our last run," "We're tapped," "We're exhausted," and "We're tired of getting up at this ungodly hour!" YES, all of that goes through our minds, while running from time to time, and will go through yours! However, once our run is over, we feel exhilarated, full of energy, and proud of ourselves because we did it "just one more time."

We promise you that if you rush into your newfound love of running that you will burnout quickly. We also promise you that you will have days when you feel like we described above, as if it will be your last run ever. On those days, you will literally need to dig down deep and say to yourself, "I can do this one more time. I'm worth it!" And, guess what ladies, you will do it one more time, and next time after that, and next time after that...

The most important promise we can make to you is that the gains you will receive by starting small will be priceless. Remember to always consult with your doctor before beginning any exercise regimen.

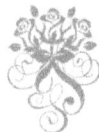

TIP

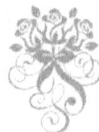

Write out your running schedule
in 4 to 6 week increments. While keeping your ultimate goal in mind, these short increments will give you a feeling of success.

Yolanda "Smelling the Roses" on Start Small

Please truly grasp the meaning of these two words "Start Small." Starting small will lead to **BIG** accomplishments. Each small goal is leading to a big prize. For me, approximately every 3-6 months, brought a new and exciting change. I never went by the scale. I knew I just loved the way I was feeling. I couldn't wait to see the progress each month. I was so glad I started small. Starting small made such a difference in my progress. It is easy to get caught up in wanting something so fast and so bad. As we all know, good things come to those who wait.

With each small goal that I accomplished, a new reward was granted to me that I could visually see within 3-6 months. I did not go into this expecting so many small benefits to be gained. One of the habits of successful people is to start small and that was comforting for me to hear. I began to visualize each few months what the next few months would bring as well as how I would look and feel. I was my own coach revising and revamping and mostly, evaluating what I could do better each time. I was creating a road map to my success.

You may feel that starting small will take you the long route, but actually, your body will respond to small steps sooner than you think. Your body will tell you when it is ready to increase the pace and it will feel comfortable doing so; then you will know to move it up to the next level.

Keep in mind that as you start small you, too, are in the beginning state of creating your very own roadmap to your success. You will have to do some re-evaluating, make changes and revamping to the small goals you have set. Don't give up and get frustrated because that is what most people will do. Set yourself up to succeed and don't worry, you will perfect the process and gain a lot of knowledge along the way and then you, too, will be able to help others.

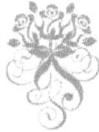

TIP

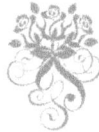

To make a run seem easier, do something such as birdwatch, count the trees — anything fun to distract your attention from running.

Itarsha "Smelling the Roses" on Start Small

Starting small to me used to be senseless. Why start small, when you can just dive in and take the bull by the horns? That used to be my philosophy. Boy was I wrong! I don't know about you, but I went through years of starting too "big" to only end up ditching everything a few days or weeks later. It was just too overwhelming to think about this large task much less commit to it.

So I tried to approach running differently, so that I would stick to it, and it worked. My whole point in telling you this is to let you know that Rome wasn't built in a day or even in a month! Ladies, you have to start small, if you want to make running part of your life. You are going to really need to take your journey one day at a time, like I did. Trust me, I know you might want to jump out there and "run" yourself to your ideal weight and size in no time, but if you do, I guarantee, you will experience burnout. Those times of wanting to quit will come and go with you, as they did and still do with me. Ladies, remember to talk yourself "through" it and not "out of it." Do you want to know the good thing? Those times of wanting to quit will come far less as you progress. So what this all boils down to and what I want to stress is to please start small. Even if it means that you change just one thing a month! Always remember that a little change is always better than no change at all. Also remember, that a little can go a long way. So, come on ladies, we are changing our lives one small change at a time.

Now that you have made the commitment and set your goals...LETS GET STARTED!

Chapter 4

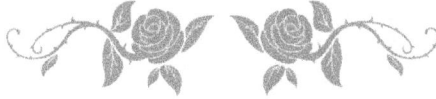

WHAT TO WEAR

Shoes

It's very imperative that you wear the proper footwear to avoid injuries. Improper footwear can cause pain in your legs, hips, thighs, calves, knees, and other parts of your body. We did extensive research and found it suggested to change your footwear every three months if running outside and every three to six months if running a mixture of on the streets and on the treadmill.

We both have made huge mistakes of not changing out of our footwear in a timely manner. We primarily run outside and should be regularly changing our footwear at the three-month mark. In the beginning, we would run with the same footwear for six months or more. As a result, both of us experienced various conditions such as chin splints, aggravated ingrown toe nail, hip pain, tight calves, ankle pain, and knee pain.

Ladies, you need to research the best running shoes for you. As an option, you may visit a podiatrist. They can give you an idea of what type of feet you have, your instep, and often times measure your gait (your style of running) which will enhance your knowledge on what running shoes are best for you. There are also some athletic stores that specialize in running gear and running shoes. Some of these stores will allow you to run a few minutes on a treadmill to video tape your running style in order to recommend a running shoe for you. You can research the Internet for a store like this near you.

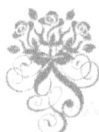

TIP

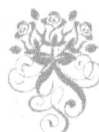

If you land hard on your heels
you will wear down your running shoes quicker than someone who runs on the ball of their feet or who is a mid-strike runner. You will need to buy new running shoes more often.

Attire

So you are ready to hit the road with your new running shoes, your eight-year-old sweats, stretched out gym shorts or the daisy dukes you found on sale, right? WRONG! Ladies, we are so sorry to burst your bubble, but those items are not going to work for running. Wearing the proper running attire is almost as important as wearing the correct running shoes. Even wearing the wrong bra, panties, and socks can hinder your run. There is nothing worse than getting five minutes into your run and your breasts are bouncing too much, your panties are rising on one or both sides and your socks are sliding down into your shoe. Ugh! This may sound comical, but seriously ladies, it's no laughing matter when you find yourself in that situation. Wearing the wrong fitness attire is the most uncomfortable feeling imaginable.

When we began our journey to becoming runners, we dressed improperly. We wore all the wrong clothing. We had no idea how to dress. Our first winter as runners, we wore sweatpants. If it was really cold, we would wear a pair of cotton stretch pants underneath our sweatpants or two pair of sweatpants. We would also wear one or two long sleeve shirts underneath a sweatshirt. The temperature would drop to 30 or 20 degrees on some mornings and we thought the warmer we dressed the better. However, the extra clothing made running difficult. We couldn't move, and we became overheated before we reached our first mile. Truly, we don't want you to experience this horrible feeling. We want to save you from that uncomfortable situation we experienced.

On cold days, your goal is to stay as dry and warm as possible. It's reported that you can lose 40% of your heat from your head, so it's important to keep it covered. Keeping your neck, ears, and hands covered will also aid in keeping your body warm. Your clothing should provide the perfect balance of trapping some air to keep you warm, and yet be able to release enough vapor or heat to avoid overheating.

After conducting, a little research, we found what worked for us. On cold days, we wear Dryfit or compression fabric for our tops, bottoms, thermo hat, gloves, and a handkerchief tucked under our bra strap for those runny nose days. Our attire has a mock neck top, which help keeps our necks warm. When the weather is extremely cold, we wear turtlenecks under our attire to cover our necks for additional warmth.

We live in North Carolina and 17 degrees is the coldest temperature we have run in since we started running in this particular state. We have had some windy days, but very few. We strongly suggest taking the temperature and wind chill factor for your part of the country into consideration, when researching cold weather attire. The reason: It may be necessary for you to layer, or be very specific with your choice of fabric if you are running below 17 degrees and possibly at times with wind. Worst case scenario, when it's too cold, we recommend hitting the treadmill.

Summer attire is pretty easy. We find that wearing basic aerobic-type workout pants that come to the knee or just above the knee and a tank top or tee shirt (not to tight or too loose) works well. A sweat band is helpful and again, a handkerchief tucked inside your bra strap to wipe away any sweat on your face as you run.

For some reason we have never run in running shorts. We are both very tall with long legs. We are pretty sure if we did, we would feel like our bottoms were being exposed with every bounce. Also, the weather will be very hot on some days, so ladies, please do not wear your shorts too short and expose too much. Please keep in mind that shorts do rise.

It's very different running with heat and humidity. The change to a hot climate can affect how you run in the winter vs. summer. You may find that you run a little slower due to the heat and humidity, but you will adjust. This is one of the reasons why we choose to run early in the mornings, before going to work, since it is the coolest time of a hot day. Please do your research to find what running attire is best for you.

Fitness attire, along with running shoes, is an investment that you must make. If you are going to do this and do this right, sacrifice ladies and invest in your health! You are so worth it!

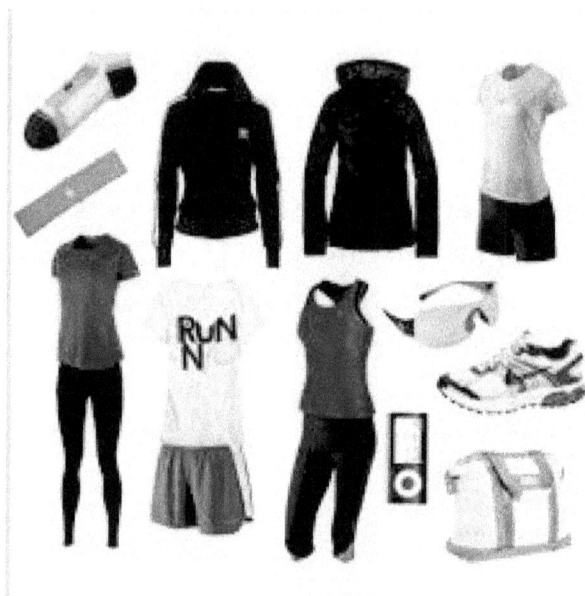

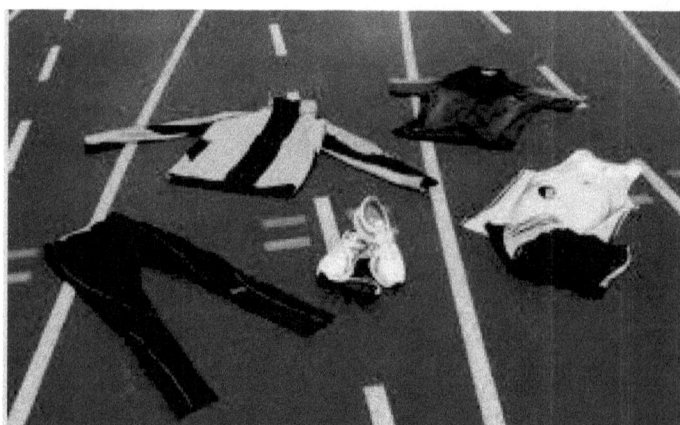

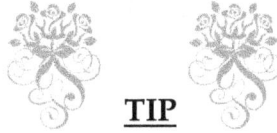

TIP

Dress the Part

Though a cotton tee shirt may work in the summer months, it may not be as comfortable as you would like it to be while running. If possible, wear running gear year around. You will find that the lightweight material of real running gear feels more comfortable against your skin the more you sweat.

Itarsha "Smelling the Roses" on What To Wear

I can tell you some funny stories about this topic. In the beginning, naturally, I wore what I had in my closet and drawers. I didn't have very much to wear outside to run in, so I wore what I had. We began walking in the spring, which wasn't too bad in terms of what I had to wear. I didn't want to spend very much on additional workout clothes, so the tee shirts, tank tops, and $3.99 stretch pants that I found on sale, worked just fine. Those inexpensive items became my wardrobe of choice for those spring and summer walks. As the colder months approached, I began wearing those same stretch pants under a pair of sweats or track pants. Sometimes two pair of stretch pants! Along with that, I would have on a turtleneck, two to three sweat shirts, a sweat jacket, a couple of hats, and a few pair of gloves. I had the nerve to begin running in that attire. Well, sort of running, because moving in all of those clothes was a challenge. It was February 2009, when we began running one full mile without stopping. Boy were we tired and hot when we finished!

When I had on several layers of bulky clothing, I felt weighed down and restricted. I would begin to sweat and get overheated. I couldn't remove anything, while I was in the middle of my run, because I was afraid of catching pneumonia, if I did.

I said all that to say, don't make the same mistake I made. I'm here to save you from that. Once I purchased real "running gear" it made my time out in the cold climate much easier and more enjoyable. Even running in the warmer weather was better in real running gear because the clothes are lighter and less restricted.

Like we previously mentioned and pictured above, there are several types of running gear that you can purchase. In the beginning, you might be hesitant because it's pricey stuff. However, you can't put a price on your health, so ladies make the investment, because you are investing in yourself.

Yolanda "Smelling the Roses" on What to Wear

After wearing all the wrong things and being uncomfortable as my thighs would rub together while walking, I realized I needed to spend some money on a summer and winter wardrobe to help. Fitted shirts (not tight) and knee length stretch pants, really worked the best for me in the summer, especially due to the fact that I had big thighs. And in the beginning, yes, my thighs were rubbing together. I hated that feeling. It made me more determined to lose weight to stop the rubbing.

I remember a time when I was walking down the hall at work, and as I was walking, my thighs made a noise in the pants I had on as they were rubbing together. Well, there was another person walking ahead of me, and they turned around without verbally saying, but having the facial expression of saying, "What in the heck is that noise?" I politely said, "Don't worry. It's just my thighs rubbing together." My big thighs did not keep me from becoming a runner.

I found great pants to run in that made my run more comfortable. It makes such a difference to run in gear that slightly holds things in place. If you are running outside, people see you, and I don't like to have panty lines showing. I prefer to run in a cotton support thong.

A great support bra is so needed. I can't stress that enough. I wear a support bra and snug sports bra to keep my breast from bouncing. It's not a good feeling to feel your chest moving while running and it's just not good to do period. Keep in mind, there is a difference between a support bra and a sports bra. You would wear both. No one needs to see your nipples and the actual shape of your breasts. For your comfort, your breasts need all the support they can get. That goes from small breasts to big breasts. When I am running, I am sweating like someone poured a bucket of water all over me. And, it is important to me that, while I am running, no one can see through my bra, shirt, or pants.

We have all seen runners, as we're driving down the road that make us say, "OH MY, REALLY!" Why in the world would someone wear that while running? I just knew if I was going to have my big self out there running, I was going to look like I had some sense. When I would see larger people running that wore appropriate attire, no matter how big they were I would say, "Good for them getting fit."

Big, medium, or small, no matter what size you are, if you are going to be out there running, you must represent the best image you can because, guess what, you are a role model for many people driving by in their cars. I promise you a stranger will be proud of you!

When I finally got the right summer and winter attire, although I was comfortable and very motivated in my fitted clothing, honestly, I was a little unhappy with how my body looked in the clothing. Don't get me wrong the fitted clothing felt great, and I felt like a true runner in it. Keeping it real: When you put on fitted clothing, you can see all your rolls, bumps, and lumps, and I had a lot of them. When I started, I was wearing loose fitted clothing that would not show all the rolls, bumps, and lumps. In my new gear and with my new attitude, I knew I was on the path to change all that, and I did!

No matter how big or small you are, the fitted clothing is always going to make you feel better than the loose fitting T-shirts and sweat pants. Each month, my attire began to look better on me as my body changed. It was amazing to me to see this change! Buying running gear can be a lot of fun. Picking out nice colors and just feeling good in that clothing will keep you motivated.

As for the shoes we mentioned previously, you will have to start with your doctor to find out what kind of feet you have and go from there. Sometimes you will see some very cute and beautiful colors on all type of shoes. Do not ever think anything will work because that is simply not true. I would love to run in shoes with beautiful colors of the rainbow, but the ones for me are not colorful. They are comfortable and do what they do to keep me running for a long time.

Preparation and Organization

Preparing and organizing your running gear ahead of time will not only save you time, but can also help you mentally prepare for your run. It comes down to organization: The more you have laid out and prepared, then the quicker you can get out the door. And the quicker you can get out the door, the less time you have to contemplate or come up with an excuse to skip your run.

We find that being ready for the next day or the entire week makes it easier to be on this journey. We find the more you have ready to go the night before, if you are a morning runner, equals a few more minutes of sleep in the morning and that is worth everything. If you are an evening runner, or if you go to the gym to run, the same applies. When you get home from work, you want to be able to just put on your gear and head out the door, before those evening distractions start to creep up. If you go to the gym, have that bag packed and put it in your car or by the door. Ladies, you can't ever be too prepared or overly organized for your run. Being unprepared cannot only cost you time, but can also distract you mentally and throw off your motivation. If you have to run around the house to find this, or find that, and you can't locate something or it's unclean, that can possibly put your head in another space. In one hot second, your motivation can disappear. Lack of preparation can also result in you being frustrated or discouraged, especially if you are on a time schedule and have other obligations to take care of after your run.

For us, we knew one would be waiting for the other. It's not fun getting a call from your running partner saying they are late, because they can't find their earphones, while you are already waiting at their door. We understand that some things cannot be prevented. It is best to get out while you have that motivation and get going as soon as your gear is on and ready. The best way to accomplish this is to be prepared and organized. Just like everything else, up to this point, preparing for your run in advance will get easier and become second nature.

Yolanda "Smelling the Roses" on Preparation And Organization

Everyone's regiment for getting organized for your morning run will be different. Being ready the night before is a big necessity for me. I have to wake up and have it all laid out ready to go from the music to the underwear. Did I do it wrong in the beginning? Yes, I did. I did not set my alarm clock correctly, could not find my gloves, hat, etc. In the beginning, I learned that it was best for me to lay out all my running gear the evening before, so I could enjoy the rest of my evening and still be prepared for my early morning run.

When you think about preparation and organization in addition to your running gear, remember it goes for any other areas of your life that can best prepare you for a great start to your day. I am a big list person—listing out what I am going to do on the daily, helps me to really stay focused.

In addition to being a list person, I am also very analytical down to the smallest detail. It is so nice to have a hobby to analyze instead of people...lol! So, if anyone is analyzing you too much, then tell them to get a hobby.

Once you have prepared and organized your day and/or week for your runs for so long, you will get to the point where everything is like second nature and you just do it!

Itarsha "Smelling the Roses" on Preparation And Organization

Yikes! "I didn't charge my iPod" or "Darn, I grabbed those running bottoms that are now too big and they keep sliding down." These are thoughts that went through my mind in the beginning of a run that I didn't properly prepare for ahead of time.

Ladies, let me tell you, if you don't take the small amount of time it takes to prepare and get organized for your next run, then it can cause you to be uncomfortable out there running on the road. Actually, it can mess up your entire mood. Take it from me; I've been there on more than one occasion in the past. There have been a few times when I didn't have the right gear or grabbed the wrong sneakers, but had to keep it moving out the door because Yolanda was waiting. Believe me, the regret of not being prepared will stay with you for your entire run.

Now, I prepare the night before. I actually start preparing at the end of each run by charging my iPod immediately before hitting the shower. You will find that it's so much more enjoyable when you are prepared vs. unprepared when hitting the road.

Get Up!

If you decide that early morning runs fit your lifestyle, we cannot stress enough the importance of the phrase "GET UP." This is the hardest and most difficult part, and it will never get easy. Physically, mentally, and sometimes emotionally, your body will fight it, but the good thing is once you "GET UP," you are halfway there!

The drive and motivation for you to get up is going to come from the feeling you will get from running consistently (even in the first week). The endorphins you release and the energy you will have throughout the day will be the best feeling you will ever experience. It's an instant feeling of satisfaction. Your run is done and the entire day is yours. Now that's a wonderful feeling!

We have to admit, there are a few sacrifices that come along with getting up so early, but the benefits in the long run far outweigh the small sacrifices involved.

You may ask, "What are the sacrifices?" Three days a week we get up at the crack of dawn, at times while everyone in the house is still asleep, heck most of the world is still asleep! It's especially hard when it's the middle of January and its 20 degrees outside those doors. We have to check the weather, so that we dress appropriately or decide to run at the gym, if it's raining.

When on vacation, we don't sleep in, we get up early to run, and often before everyone gets up. We have to make certain we still run on vacation. That's right! We said while on vacation, or we will lose some of our endurance and gains, which does nothing more than make the very next run tougher.

Once our morning runs are complete, it's like euphoria; it's such a peaceful, happy feeling to know we've done something great for ourselves. Something no one else can do for us. We did something special for ourselves first thing in the morning, which fills us up to give to our families, friends, and jobs for the day.

What's amazing is that the above motivating factors are just icing on the cake! Additional and more long-term benefits of running are:

1) Cardiovascular health

2) Osteoporosis prevention

3) Regulates blood pressure

4) Achieve ideal body weight

5) Increased muscle tone & endurance

6) Cellulite reduction

7) Relieves stress

8) Mental clarity & focus

And also, if it's your desire to fit into that size 6 dress, guess what? You can achieve all the above benefits without taking a weight loss pill! Now what's better than that? So girl GET UP!!

Itarsha "Smelling the Roses" on Get Up!

On the morning of my runs, the first thing I do is turn on the television to check the weather because I need to be comfortably dressed throughout my run. Like we briefly mentioned before, and trust me when I say, the worst thing to be is too "hot" or too "cold" during a 5 mile run! Unfortunately, I've been both at one time or another, and I was pretty miserable during those times. I live in Raleigh, North Carolina, and there is a period during the year when the weather can vary drastically from day-to-day. Usually it's when it's coming out of the summer, or going into the summer. During those times, I never assume what the weather will feel like outdoors. I will look at the weather and prepare the night before. I still always peek at the weather again the morning of my run. I don't put away my summer gear until we are well into the fall or almost winter.

Same for my winter gear. It's not put away until the end of spring.

Like we discussed under, the Preparation & Organization chapter, preparing what gear I'm wearing to run in the night before is vital to me. Every now and then, the weatherman may be a little off, as it pertains to the temperature, and if that happens, I usually will need to only change a long sleeve to a short sleeve or vice versa. Everything else will be prepared. Getting up out of my warm bed to run is a tad bit easier when I'm prepared.

My family members weren't quite sold on the idea that I would be getting up to run on a regular basis at first. However, once they noticed time and time again, week after week I was getting up, getting dressed and out the door like clockwork, my commitment began to sink in. About two or three months into my morning runs I could tell in little ways I was being supported for my efforts. Little things like not being disturbed when I turned in early and finding that my workout clothes and gear were given a designated area, showed me that my commitment was being noticed. Those were small ways my family told me they were on board with my journey.

To this day, while on vacation, I always get up and head straight to the hotel gym to run on the treadmill. I check-in with everyone I'm vacationing with the night before to find out what the next day plans are, so I know what time I need to get up, run, and get back in time. My family and friends are now used to me doing this. Again, prepping the night before will help so that you are not fumbling around the hotel room for your gear.

Trust me, you will get the stink eye from whomever you are vacationing with, if you do this.

The drive and determination to "GET UP" and "GET OUT" was never part of my daily regimen. Before my love for running came about, people around me had to slowly adjust. So ladies, remember to give your family time to adjust to your new commitment to running. I promise you, they will adjust as long as they see you are determined to "GET UP!"

Yolanda "Smelling the Roses" on Get Up!

I am not going to even lie. Some mornings, it is very hard to get up, especially when you are a beginner at running. I asked myself "how do I do it?" Well, the best answer I can come up with is it's because I am doing something for me that will make me a better person. I also can say I have seen the results and I like them!

As soon as the alarm goes off, I rise up quickly. Hitting snooze is not an option. Get up and it will pay off! This takes discipline and at times a total mindset. You have to be very dedicated to your goal. Knowing the temperature outside the morning of your run is 27 degrees, can be an excuse, if you let it be one. On average I need at least 6-7 hours of sleep. This makes me have to turn in early in the evenings. For me, running is much better when I have the proper rest I need. It is amazing to me how I can be a little tired when I get up and get started, and by the time I am finished I am so energetic that being tired is an afterthought.

Before long, at times your body will want to get up way before your mind tells it to, because you are training your body to do that. Really, you are training your mind and your body. When you step out that door, your mind and body will be in sync and work together to get the job done.

What To Eat Before And After Running

Since we are not certified dieticians or nutritionists, you will have to perform research, talk with your doctor, or see a nutritionist, whichever will work best for you when it comes to your post-run meals. We can tell you what we choose to eat after we run. Since we prefer to run first thing in the morning what works for us is to choose not to eat until after our run is over. We always have a 32oz. container of water waiting for us to drink directly following our run. Drinking lots of water is essential to rehydrating yourself after and sometimes during your run.

After our run, we usually eat foods containing carbohydrates such as a piece of fruit, toast, bagel, oatmeal, or yogurt. These are foods that will instantly refuel your body. An hour or so later, you may want that big protein breakfast and that is okay. We also make sure we take a daily multi-vitamin.

The above are just suggestions and by no means meant to be set in stone. Everyone is different. Some people feel the need to eat a little something before their run or drink water midway through their run. Absolutely do what your body craves!

We can't stress enough for you to do your own research, or seek advice from your doctor, or a nutritionist to educate yourself on what will work best for you and your body's individual needs. We both eat differently. What works for one does not work necessarily for the other. There are so many resources today, and it should be easy for you to find something that works for you.

Itarsha "Smelling the Roses" on What To Eat Before And After Running

This is a touchy topic, so I'm not going to go into it too much. However, I do want to put out there that I love to eat. I love the way food tastes, the way it smells, and the way it looks. Though I don't deprive myself, I try to be cautious of what I eat in general. However, the operative word here is "try." I usually eat what I want with portion control, and I have always tried to eat like this each day. I'm not extremely strict on myself, so some days it works and some days it doesn't work. The good thing is that on the days that my eating is sort of *off* I don't let it bother me. Like I said before, being committed to running first and foremost will make all other fitness goals fall into place. This goes for eating, too!

Personally, I don't feel good running with something on my stomach. On one occasion, I ate half of a banana, and on another occasion, I ate half of a protein bar and both times my stomach felt uncomfortable during my run. Both times, I tried to eat before a run, because I ran later than usual, so I thought I should eat a little something since it was later in the morning. I only tried twice to eat before a run and due to those experiences, I think I will just do what's been working for me, which is to run on an empty stomach. It's just a personal preference for me to eat after I complete my run. I actually am not really that hungry after I run. However, I eat because I know I need to feed my body after putting the stress of running five miles onto it.

Whatever you decide to do for your nutritional needs, before and after you run, make sure you do what's deemed best for your fitness goals, your health, and your body.

Yolanda "Smelling the Roses" on What To Eat Before And After Running

When I began this journey, I researched a few topics of what to eat before and after running. I found many different views on this topic. At first, I tried to eat a little something such as a few sips of a protein shake, a banana, or a granola bar. I am not saying these items are the right things to eat. It's just what I've tried. After trying some of these foods in the morning prior to my run, I found that I would have a slight cramp in my side after running a ½ mile. I noticed with taking a few sips of water or a protein shake, I would unfortunately create a need to have to urinate not long after beginning to run. And, that's not a fun feeling to have to go urinate while in the middle of your run.

As you have read, you now know that I am an early morning runner. I found the thing that works better for me is to not to eat or to drink prior to running. After my run, I drink a lot of water. Then approximately one to two hours after my run, I eat a small breakfast, like yogurt, cereal, oatmeal, or a protein shake. I did not realize in the beginning how important it was to really watch what you eat, as it relates to your daily calorie intake. It is important that your running works hand and hand with a proper caloric intake in order to achieve the best results. Please do your research and find what works best for you. It may take some time to figure out what is a good balance for you. Everyone is different and what I do for me may not work for you. Many people cannot have dairy and are Gluten-free, etc. and there are so many allergies to take into consideration. I am one that suffers from food allergies. It is not like a one size fits all type of thing. You will have to experiment and come to the best conclusion for you.

Chapter 5

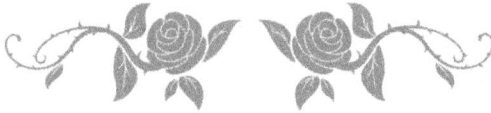

SAFETY

We cannot stress enough how important it is to find a partner that will be there for you through the thick and thin of running. Having a partner run with you is a large part of being safe and staying safe, when it comes to safety overall. If you can't find a dedicated partner, then join a running group. Running is much more enjoyable when you are not distracted and preoccupied with having to look over your shoulder every five minutes because you are running alone. Don't get us wrong, when running with a partner and/or group or not, you must ALWAYS stay alert, but with a partner or group, you can act as a team while on your run.

In addition to having a partner or running with a group, we recommend purchasing a small can of pepper spray or mace. Many stores carry a small three-inch size convenient for runners. We found our pepper spray at a local firearms store. You may check in your area for a store that sells pepper spray or mace, or you may purchase a can online. You need to look for one with a clip, so it can clip on to your waist or shirt. We clip ours to our shirt near the collarbone for easy access.

Running with a reflector vest on is a must. It makes you 20 times more visible to anyone walking or driving. These vests can be found in the camping section of a sporting goods store.

Now that you have your partner, mace, pepper spray, and your reflective vest, you are in the best position to be safe while on your run. One of the best safety measures that do not involve spending money is to ALWAYS be aware of your surroundings. Being aware and following your instincts is vital. There have been a few times we can recall seeing things that looked out of place ahead of us while running. These are things like:

1) an untied dog
2) unfamiliar cars parked on the side of the road, and
3) other runners or walkers, we've never seen before

In these situations, we've made the decision to follow our instinct to turn and run in another direction. Deciding to change directions was to avoid what may or may not have been. We have never regretted diverting from our route when we were uneasy about our surroundings, because we never gave it a second thought. Deciding to change directions was and will always be an automatic reaction when and if anything at all looks out of place. Use your intuition and go with your gut! Always, always, always choose safety first when in doubt!

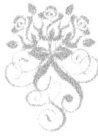

TIP

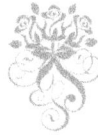

While running with music,
keep the volume down and stick to familiar routes that offer good visibility, so you can see what and whom is around you.

Yolanda "Smelling the Roses" on Safety

Well get ready because you're gonna hear this from your spouse, boyfriend, friends, and/or family: "**It's not safe to run out there.**" You will always have many that will be concerned and with good reason. For us, everyone close to us is aware of all the precautions we take—the pepper spray, the reflective vest, etc. That is very comforting to them.

You want to be sure to reassure your friends and loved ones that you are as safe as you can be while on a run. Be open to any suggestions they have to offer. Running with loud music makes you have to be extra cautious. You can let yourself get so into the music that you cannot hear a car. I have heard of many runners that were hit because they were turning or going across the street without looking. I have had to run by myself plenty of times, and I always put my safety first by making sure the sun is up. Sometimes I don't run with music in order to be more alert. Honestly, I do not take any chances when it comes to safety. I guess I've watched America's Most Wanted, CSI, and other crime shows too many times. I am ready for whatever, always!

Running with a small pouch around your waist may work for some. This will allow you to carry additional items of protection. We will always advise you to do research and be smart.

Itarsha "Smelling the Roses" on Safety

The very first thing I would like to say is your safety ALWAYS comes first! There have been times that I felt a little unsafe or uneasy while running. This didn't happen often, but the times I've felt this way are times I can remember because the incidents really shook me up.

One warm morning we were running very early and since it was a warm morning, it may have been summer time. During the summer months, we begin our runs earlier than during the rest of the year to beat the heat. Often we are running when it's still dark or what may be considered the dawn of the morning. On this particular morning, I was a little way in front of Yolanda and began to approach this guy who was waiting for someone outside of a house. Though he seemed to be waiting on another person so that they could go for a walk, I didn't know that at the time, and I was getting closer to approaching him while he stood there, alone in the dark, while he watched me get closer to him. I had never seen him out there previously, and I began to feel uneasy. I pulled out my pepper spray and held it tightly in my hand, as I ran closer towards him. Fortunately, he and his friend were walkers. I felt kind of silly when his friend came out, and they waved and started walking in the other direction. Though they meant me no harm, and all was well, I was still prepared to defend myself, if it came to it. Then, there was a time a dog actually ran up on me, and before I knew it, I pepper-sprayed him! Needless to say he turned and ran away never to be seen by me again.

Yolanda and I run with music, so we depend on our eyes, our feelings, and each other to observe when something isn't right. I never second guess myself, if the situation doesn't look or feel right, I act. Yolanda runs at a different pace than I do. She runs at a comfortable pace for herself, as I do. Oftentimes, I'm in front of her. As I mentioned earlier, we run in the mornings and sometimes it's still dark outside. Our runs cover so much area, including running blocks and turning corners. We also run through three different neighborhoods, and at one point, we ran along the paved roads in a golf course. When it's dark, I always wait for Yolanda by running in circles or running back and forth, until she reaches me, or is within eyesight. I just feel better knowing that she made it around the corner or from one neighborhood to another. If I see something that doesn't look right, I turn around and slow down for her, or change directions, and she does the same. We never question each other when this happens, we just follow what the other is doing and know there is a reason for it. More than likely if one of us detours from the route, it's for our safety in some shape, form, or fashion.

Keep It Clean

Ladies, we hope this doesn't offend anyone. Please know that this is not our intention. You are an adult, and of course we know, that you know how to keep yourself clean, so in NO WAY are we talking about this to insult you, so please take into consideration the advice that we are giving. If you are on this journey, you will quickly learn the real meaning of sweating because you will sweat a lot! At the beginning of your journey, and as it was for us, you won't realize how much water can pour off your body until you run. We had to test and try different techniques to keep the sweat under control, so we say "keep it clean" to those of you who may find yourselves in that same condition.

Sweating is a great thing. It's actually healthy to sweat! However, it's not as easy to control as one may think! We sweat tremendously, and after the first mile, sweat is pouring down our faces. We sweat so much we can literally ring out our clothes and make a puddle, after we run. We keep a small bandana or handkerchief tucked somewhere on us to wipe as we run. As soon as we wrap up our run, we get out of our clothes right away. We can't even venture out to run a quick errand after we run, because our clothes are soaking wet. There is no way we would be caught in a store or anywhere that way. Trust us, it's not cute at all.

What we want to also stress here is please, please do not make the mistake of thinking you can wear the same running clothing the next time without washing them. Both in the winter and summer months have a fresh clean set of running attire waiting for your next run. Yes, it can be expensive to go out and buy the proper attire to have for each day, but it is worth the sacrifice to keep you clean, organized, and prepared.

We both sweat so much, we can't even sit on our car seats after a run without soaking the seat. We have to line the car seats with a seat cover or towel. Bacteria loves a sweaty environment, so get out of your running clothing as soon as you can and take that great shower you have earned!

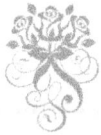

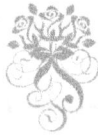

TIP
Shower immediately after running.
Bacteria loves sweat! Also, pollen from the air and trees can settle on your clothes, hair, and face which can trigger allergies.

Itarsha "Smelling the Roses" on Keep It Clean

The amount of sweat that can excrete from your body will always remain a mystery, until you become a runner. I never in my wildest dreams thought I could sweat as much as I do. I used to think I didn't sweat much and that's because I didn't.

After running, I am covered from the top of my head to the bottom of my socks in sweat, and it doesn't feel or smell good.

I quickly found something else out about my severe sweating during my runs. I can't wear certain colored running pants because the sweat comes through a lot in the middle of my pants. Yikes! How embarrassing this was when it happened on more than one occasion! It didn't click at first that grays and browns weren't my friend when it comes to running pants. However, it didn't take long for me to figure it out! I am very strategic now when purchasing pants to run in. Black is always the safe way to go for me. So don't be alarmed when something similar to this happens to you because it comes with the territory. No worries, because just like I did, you will find the best way to manage those types of problems. This is a small thing in the grand scheme of your journey. So with no pun intended: Ladies, don't sweat the small stuff.

Yolanda "Smelling the Roses" on Keep It Clean

We may sound redundant on this point. I cannot believe how wet with sweat I am after a run. I have to constantly wipe my face. After the first ten minutes I am already sweating. We just want you to be prepared for it. I did not even know I could sweat so much until I became a runner. All of the benefits I get from running and sweating are worth it.

As far as I am concerned you CANNOT re-wear any first and second layer running gear the next day without washing it! No, you CANNOT wear the same socks two days in a row.

Your feet sweat and you too will discover many parts of your body are sweating that you did not know could. It is really good for your body to release those toxins by sweating. To help me keep it clean, I chose to buy several pieces of running clothing essential to my success. It was an investment, but a good one. I have fresh running clothing for each day. On one of your running days in the middle of your run it can pour down rain all of sudden and when you get home not only are your clothes, hair and body wet, but your shoes are soaked. Well, those wet shoes can smell if they do not properly dry. Having another pair of running shoes as back up is always a good plan that you can use while the others are properly drying out. You do not want to have smelly shoes the next day and have to run in them. I am told I am the queen of organization, well I used that skill to help me save time as it relates to preparing clean running gear each day and look forward to helping you do this to.

Breathing While Running

Running and breathing go hand and hand. In order to be successful in building endurance and stamina you will need to breathe properly. Taking in enough air during your run is essential for this to happen. We both have different running styles and each of us run the way that is comfortable for us individually. This also relates to our breathing, so since we run differently, our breathing is different, too.

Our running pace controls our breathing. We know we are running too fast, if we can't breathe, or it becomes difficult to breathe. You should always be in control of your breathing. You should not be gasping for air as you run. If you are, please slow down. It's not a good idea to sacrifice how much air you are taking into your lungs, or sacrifice how comfortable you are able to breathe for speed. Our breathing changes throughout our run, as we change our pace as well as when going up or down hills. Once our pace is under control our breathing follows. We just recommend doing what works for you and makes you feel comfortable. The best advice we can give is to please take the time to research different breathing methods for runners online.

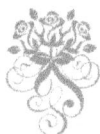

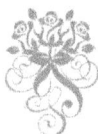

TIP

Your mouth is larger than your nostrils,
so it's more effective at taking in oxygen. Also, keeping your mouth open, keeps your face more relaxed, which makes it easier to breathe deeply.

Itarsha "Smelling the Roses" on Breathing While Running

Breathing is easy, right? Breathe in, breathe out. That's all there is to it. Well not exactly when it comes to running. When I first began to run, I felt like I would have a heart attack after about a mile! What I wasn't doing was breathing correctly for the pace I was running. I wasn't taking in enough air, and therefore, I felt like I was going to pass out.

One thing I realize is that my breathing pattern varies throughout my run. This is something that I didn't pay attention to in the beginning. However, changing my breathing pattern is what helps me. I have to change the amount of air I take in, how fast and how often, based upon the pace and my distance. Since we all are different and have different lung capacities, this will vary from person to person.

The right breathing pattern was one of the biggest trial and error areas during my journey. Just like me, you'll get it right. Practice makes perfect with breathing and running.

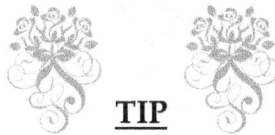

TIP

New runner tip:
Focus on going further before going faster.

Yolanda "Smelling the Roses" on Breathing While Running

Nobody had to tell me how to breathe...lol. I was not trying to have a cardiac arrest on the side of the road. If I could not breathe, I would just slow down until I was able to run at a breathable pace. What I can tell you is as my body adjusted to the breathing, I was able to improve my pace and increase my distance. Getting my breathing right took time and patience. Some days my breathing was loud and other days it was really loud.

When the thought of running five miles crossed my mind prior to this journey, I would have said there is no way I can even breathe enough to make it 1/4 of a mile or even make it up a hill without losing my breath. I just paced myself so my breathing stays under control. As my endurance got stronger by breathing got better.

Chapter 6

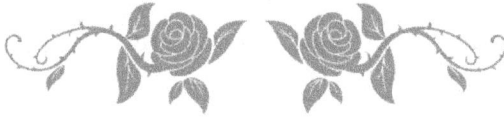

HAVE MULTIPLE RUNNING ROUTES

We decided it was less repetitive and more interesting to map out a few different running routes. We were so glad we had that option. We had routes with lots of little hills, big hills, and huge hills. Of course, since we were alternating going to each other's house each day, we would indeed run in a different neighborhood, since we were starting at a different house each time. We actually had a couple of routes for each of our neighborhoods.

Having more choices in routes will be helpful for you and will truly break the monotony. You may look forward to one over the other for whatever reason. However, you'll find you can appreciate the change in scenery that comes with each route.

Changing your route is good for your legs as well. Depending on the route, and whether it has more or less hills or changes from concrete to asphalt, the change will work different muscles in your legs.

We began to know what routes had potential stray dogs and knew we had to be visually and audibly cautious, as we ran through those areas. We also had routes with a fan club of cars that would be cheering us on as we passed. So ladies, get in your car and map out those routes and make it fun!

Itarsha "Smelling the Roses" on Multiple Running Routes

As you can already tell, I love to run, but I must admit, it can get boring, if I don't make the run interesting with some great music and of course, changing up my route from time-to-time. Yolanda and I virtually had a different route to run every other run because we designed it that way. I really don't have to have that much of a change, but it's refreshing sometimes for any type of change.

Let me tell you a little bit about hills...they are a beast! No matter how experienced of a runner I am, or how long I've been running, a hill is still a hill. And to be frank, I really don't like them. I think one of our routes has a combination of 9 big and small hills! Ugh!

However, on the flip side, do you want to know the good thing about hills? They make me feel stronger and on top of the world. Once I conquer them, the rest of my run is gravy. I hope my feelings about hills do not discourage you from running them. Yes, they are challenging and sometimes grueling, but ladies, there is an upside to all of this, your legs will look amazing from running alternate routes and hills, and you will feel on top of the world, too!

Yolanda "Smelling the Roses" on Multiple Running Routes

Oh my goodness...let me say I have my favorite and not so favorite routes. The ones with the huge hills were always my least favorite. Itarsha was in front of me running all the time and seeing her ahead of me, was my biggest motivator. Those hills were rough, but I began to get better and faster getting up them. The routes with the big hills in the end gave me such a good feeling at the end of our run. Don't let the hills intimidate you. Just take your time and it will get easier and easier.

As Itarsha mentioned, it is great having multiple running routes for many reasons. It helps as a safety precaution and keeps others for knowing your routine. It helps you to see the community you live in and the area in your neighborhood. While you are on this journey, you will meet other runners, and they will ask you to run with them. It may be a situation where they ask you to join them for a run, on a track, or at the school in your neighborhood, but be open to the idea and try new things. That keeps it fun! Although I do have some routes that are my least favorite, there is something I appreciate about all of them.

Aches, Pains And Strange Feelings

Don't fool yourself into thinking you can start any form of exercise and not feel some discomfort. Your body is going to talk to you and you must listen. You have to remember your body is used to whatever your body is used to. Which means if your body is used to sitting most of the day. It wants to continue to sit most of the day, every day!

We have had our share of aches and pains. Along this journey, we have both had experiences with different body parts hurting or aching for one reason or another. For example, when you are running and your tread is just a little worn on the bottom of your shoe, it can cause your knees and/or shins discomfort. Wearing the wrong type of running shoes or running shoes with worn tread, can cause some aches and pains that may require some treatment. Always consult your physician first.

Ladies, there is no way to avoid this. Sometimes we feel pain in our lower backs, knees, calves, ankles, and heck sometimes everywhere! However, not severe enough to avoid running. We are not saying or advising you to ignore or neglect getting checked out by a doctor. However, you have to determine if it's just a sore muscle that just needs to be stretched out or if it's more serious than that, and needs to be rested or checked out. By all means, don't ignore your body; just don't let little aches scare you into quitting. Do not underestimate the power of a good chiropractor or having a monthly massage.

Running or moving your body, is just like running a car, you've got to fuel it and provide maintenance on it.

There is usually always a solution to the discomfort you may experience. Sometimes your body will ache to let you know that you need to get some rest. Rest works wonders for working out those small, minor aches. It might be that all you need is an extended pre and post stretch and that might just do the trick. We have outlined some tips below to address any aches or pains you may have during or after your runs:

1) Research to see if stretching before or after your run works for you.

2) Go see an orthopedic doctor to know what type of foot you have and any additional requirements such as a custom insert/orthotics.

3) Get a new or better shoe for your foot type.

These are just a few solutions, but just remember to never ignore any discomfort. You should always research and/or seek medical attention to find the best solution for you.

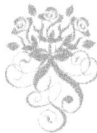

TIP

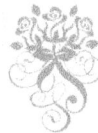

If the rubber is worn, it's time for a new pair of shoes.
More than usual aches and pains can signal that a new pair of run-ning shoes are needed.

Yolanda "Smelling the Roses" on Aches, Pains And Strange Feelings

When you first begin walking and/or running, you may experience some aches, pain and strange feelings within your thighs, abdomen, back, ankles, calves, and other areas. When we started walking, our thighs would itch after every walk for about 10 mins. We realized that it was obviously due to the blood flowing through our thighs. Itching thighs is a sign that what you are doing is working. Yay!!! You are now burning fat. We experienced this itching for about 3 months and then it stopped. Although it stopped, we knew we were still burning fat. It was now known that our thighs had adjusted to our routine and what we were doing was good! Your body will eventually give in and adjust to your new routine. We are tall women with long legs, but we still experience different aches and pains occasionally.

Some aches and pains can be avoided with proper shoes, proper form, and proper stretching. I have my favorite brand of running shoes that I love. They are perfect for me. I swear by them. It is hard to find the right running shoe, and when I did, I felt so good. In addition to proper shoes, you may need orthotics (special shoe inserts made specifically for your feet provided by a foot doctor). Once I realized that my flat feet were causing some of my knee, shin, and back pain, the orthotics amazingly alleviated the pain.

When I first started running, I would sometimes have minor aches in one of my knees and/or lower back. After going to see my physician and my orthopedic about my aches and pains a few times, I was more educated about the contributing culprits. Most of the time the culprit was the tread on my shoes. I got into a regiment of thinking that every three months I needed to change shoes, which was almost true. What I did not realize is that each time I run, I am not running on the same level of asphalt. Because of this, I was advised to check my shoes every two months for worn tread, instead of every three months.

We may be a little repetitive on this, but it will help you to know this early on. Don't let these aches and pains keep you from moving forward. Research and check with your doctor about any pains you are having and you will find there is a solution for most.

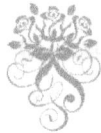

TIP

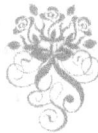

For injuries, the quicker you ice,

the faster you slow down inflammation, and the faster you begin to heal. A good way to treat injuries is by freezing water in a paper cup. Once frozen, use the exposed part of the ice to rub in a circular motion over the injury.

Itarsha "Smelling the Roses" on Aches, Pains And Strange Feelings

All I can say is that aches and pains and strange feelings come and go! The first thing you MUST get right before anything else are your running shoes. Ladies, I have two words for you: DON'T SKIMP! I know Yolanda and I touched on this when we talked about "what to wear," but it's definitely worth mentioning again. Get a good pair of running shoes and replace them as often as necessary, no matter if you don't get the recommended miles from them. One thing I can attest to is if you continue to run after your running shoes need replacing, then you will be in big trouble! I had been wearing one type of running shoe and thought they were the correct running shoes. They performed really well, but I should have replaced them way sooner than the recommended miles. I didn't notice that they needed to be replaced until my calves and shins were hurting me like crazy. Please take my advice, this is a big no-no, because it takes about two to three weeks of running in brand new shoes for the pain to go away. Fortunately, thanks to the very informative Internet, I was able to identify why I was running through my shoes so quickly and corrected the problem. Basically, what I found, is that I am a "heel striker," which means I land on my heels first. This type of stride will generally wear down a shoe quickly. It's not worth trying to save a few bucks by trying to get a couple of more weeks to a month out of your running shoes, trust me. If you do this, it will definitely cost you in the long run with aches and pain.

Injuring my hip was the scariest and most traumatic thing to happen to me from a physical standpoint. I've also had other injuries that I've had to overcome throughout my journey; some of which I still manage from day-to-day. I've broken my tibia, I've had sciatic nerve pain up and down my left leg, lower back pain, shin pain, a pinched nerve in my hip due to scoliosis curvature, and I also have a weak ankle, which aggravates me from time-to-time. My lower back pain is constant and is contributed to my life long bout with scoliosis. I do what I can to counteract my scoliosis curvature in my back from getting worse by performing a number of back exercises five days a week. Please don't misunderstand me, I will ALWAYS listen to my body and if I can't run or exercise because of pain, I don't and I won't! It's just that after so many years, I know my body extremely well. I have been able to discern when I can and cannot run or exercise.

There have been times when I've had to take a few months off from running due to some of the above aliments. During those times, I still worked out. I worked out on the elliptical machine in lieu of running. Using the elliptical machine has helped with keeping my endurance up so that when I was able to return to running, I wouldn't have a hard time getting back out there. When I know my body could run without causing more pain or injury, I tied up my sneakers, and hit the pavement and never used minor aches or soreness as an excuse not to run.

So as you can see, it's not always easy or a walk in the park for me when it comes to getting up in the morning and preparing for a run. I have to get up early enough to assess my body to make sure my body "allows" me to run each and every "run day." If my body says no, then it is no, but fortunately those times are few. It's second nature now, but has not always been that way.

Before my hip injury, I didn't take much time to assess my body before embarking on my morning run. Boy did that prove to be a huge mistake! I would run first, then wish I hadn't because XYZ would end up hurting afterward. Not just hurt, but hurt to the point where I regretted running on that particular day. That night was spent icing, heating, rolling, and resting. Ugh! Not to mention having to go to work all day sore or in pain because I didn't troubleshoot BEFORE my run. The good thing, and my body's saving grace is that we don't run on consecutive days. We run three days a week, usually Monday, Wednesday, and Friday. This schedule of alternating our running days is helpful in giving our body the break it needs on non-running days. This will be a very valuable tool and lessons, ladies.

I wrote all this to say, pain will definitely hamper a run. Over the years, I have experienced lower back pain, knee pain, ankle pain, and severe leg pain. Like I've mentioned countless times, I was born with scoliosis; it's actually severe enough to when I was a little girl, the doctors continued to urge my mother to let them operate on me. She wouldn't agree to it because she thought it might land me in a wheel chair for the rest of my life, so here I am living with it. I can walk, skip, and run on my own. So as far as I'm concerned, she made the right choice. My doctors say that I am doing the best thing for my scoliosis. GOD is good, all the time!

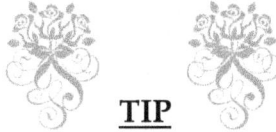

TIP

Back off at the first sign of injury.
Three to five days off is better than missing a month or two.

Hair

We briefly talked about hair prior to now by mentioning how not to use it as an excuse to "not run." We think it needs its own section because as you ladies all know, IT'S JUST THAT SERIOUS!

As you know we are minorities and have "minority hair!" We have tried every hairstyle known to mankind throughout our journey. We think we have tried everything but dreadlocks!

Contending with hair and running can easily get any woman to the point where they just want to scream. If you are a woman who doesn't happen to sweat profusely after running, consider yourself blessed! We both sweat a lot, and we do mean a lot! During our 5 mile runs, we are sweating within the first 15 minutes from top to bottom. Let us remind you that after 15 minutes, we have only run a little over 1.5 miles with 3.5 more to go! So you can imagine by the end of our run, we are drenched from head-to-toe and could both ring our clothes out, including our hair, and make a huge puddle right where we are standing.... no joke! So, you can imagine how wet our hair is afterward. It's soaking and there is little we can do about it. However, we will take wet, half-manageable hair over NOT running and going back to an unhealthy lifestyle. Ladies, which do you choose?

Yolanda "Smelling the Roses" on Hair

Honestly, I cannot offer much advice in this area, except don't let your hair keep you from being fit. I have had to truly rely on a lot of patience to help deal with this sweaty hair syndrome I live with every day. I am currently natural using no relaxer. Some days I want to slap a perm on this frizzy bush, but I do have an advantage of having a little bit of curl to my bush when it is wet. Yes, it takes me a little more work for natural hair. I would rather have that problem than having the problem of being unhealthy. When I go to the salon and get my hair nicely blow-dried out, it only lasts a day or two at the most. As soon as I run it is all gone. Unfortunately, I have a very sensitive scalp, so weaves and wigs just make my scalp itch. Solving this problem is an ongoing saga for me. However, it does not and will never keep me from my love of running.

Itarsha "Smelling the Roses" on Hair

My hair, OMG! Just the thought of what to do with it at times after a run makes me want to cringe. Right now, I wear a ponytail or bun until my relaxer starts to grow out. I relax my hair every 6 to 12 months now that I am older. I used to relax it more frequently, but it's not as strong as it used to be when I was younger. Once my relaxer starts to wear out and my bun no longer looks like a bun, then I wear lace front wigs.

Dealing with wet hair after each and every run is not fun at all. It's extremely wet, and when it dries my scalp gets dry. It's not easy at all, but what's the alternative? Well let me see: the risk of being overweight, heart disease, diabetes, and the absence of the overall wonderful feeling I get from running.

I can rock a cute hairstyle, get my hair blown out, and look great with the latest and greatest hairstyles out here, but to me my health is so much more important. I hope you don't let "hair" keep you from living your journey of becoming a runner and living the healthy lifestyle you have always dreamed of having. Ladies, the "sweaty hair" situation is so worth it in the end!

Running Events And Running Clubs

At a certain point you may find yourself interested in going online and finding new running groups, or you may want to try to run on a trail, a 5K, etc. We are used to running on asphalt as opposed to a concrete sidewalk, or if there is inclement weather, we run at the gym on a treadmill.

You may want a little bit of a change and sometimes find the need to try something different. This can help with keeping you motivated and focused on your running journey. Changing your environment can sometimes give you a fresh outlook on running and can be refreshing.

Although at this time, we don't participate in running clubs or run marathons, we have absolutely nothing against them. It takes a little more planning and a little more flexibility to participate in an organized running group or event. We are both extremely busy and it would be tough to fit a running club or marathon training plan into our already jammed packed schedule, but if you have the time, we encourage you to join. At least do your research to see what's out there, so you can readily change up your routine, when and if you ever feel like you're in a rut.

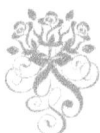

TIP

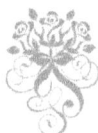

When running in a group, don't worry about keeping up with others, run at your pace.

Itarsha "Smelling the Roses" on Running Events And Running Clubs

If you can join a running club do it! I would love to be part of a running club, but really don't have the time right now. I follow a few clubs on Facebook and live vicariously through them. The thing about being part of a running club is that they run at times that do not line up with my schedule, and it will be pretty tough to enjoy being part of the club if I'm not able to run in most of the scheduled events.

I often see pictures and videos of my Facebook friends in running groups winning races or just completing them. I love seeing their smiles, as they proudly show their medals and ribbons. All of this is an inspiration to me to see them doing what they love, and getting rewarded and recognized for it. I also have gym friends that run half and whole marathons. They love telling me about their runs and where they are traveling next. I don't necessarily need to join a running group or run a marathon to stay motivated and committed to running. I love running at its core, but I commend and am very happy for people who look to these events to bring their love for running full circle.

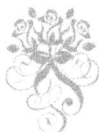

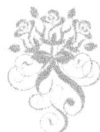

TIP
When running with others who are running with their headphones on, they may not be aware of their surroundings, so be sure you are speaking loud enough when saying you are passing on the left or right side.

Yolanda "Smelling the Roses" on Running Events And Running Clubs

Oh my goodness, I get so excited for people that take the time to share their running adventures with me. I have heard of so many fun ones. I have met people that tell me how much fun they have running on a trail with rocks and dirt. Some have shared with me a running on the beach marathon (that one sounds like fun). I am happy for their accomplishments and for them sharing that with me. I must say that I have not run in any fun events, or marathons as of yet. I may do so one day. I am so glad there are a lot of runs dedicated to wonderful charities. It is wonderful to me to know that charities can benefit from all types of runners from the beginners to the pros.

Chapter 7

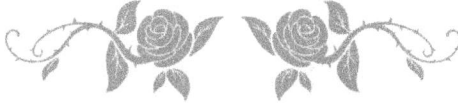

AGE MAKES NO DIFFERENCE

It is so very inspirational to see older people running or even walking. We are talking about people in their seventies and eighties doing this on a regular basis. It motivates us to know that when we get older, we can still keep our journey going for truly a lifetime. Ladies, we all know that with age, comes the pounds. It's no secret 8 out of 10 of us will begin to put on a little weight each year, after 35 years old. The other 2 out of 10 are blessed with good genes. Anyway, don't let age stop you from this wonderful journey. We began our journey in our late thirties and forties (we're not exactly spring chickens!). Research shows that people are running and loving it well into their golden years and this can include not only us, but you as well.

Do some research on what the older generation is doing to stay fit. It will truly make you say, "I have no excuse!"

Yolanda "Smelling the Roses" on Age Makes No Difference

I remember when I was younger in elementary school thinking age forty was so very old. Now that I am in my forties and my daughter is starting her own life, I feel like I have a whole new beginning. I feel better now at age 49 than I did at age 35. I'm sure some of you ladies can relate to what I am writing. For some, that feeling of having a new beginning comes at the ages of 40, 50, 60, or even older. A second or even third chance at life can come around for you at any age. What are you going to do with it?

I love to see older people out walking. It is actually motivating to me to see it, because it makes me feel that I, too, can do that when I am in my sixties and seventies. My mother keeps inspiring me as well. She has her walking regiment and it pays off for her. Her abs are better than mine and look great for her age. I have, in the past, helped others in need as a certified nursing assistant and caregiver. By doing this, I have seen clearly what the aging process can do to the body. Staying active helps.

At the end of the day, walking, jogging, running, dancing, or just moving is inspirational! Heck, do it all! For some, this book is about **Running and Smelling the Roses**, and for others that do not find it easy to run, find a way to walk or **Move and Smell the Roses!**

Itarsha 'Smelling the Roses" on Age Makes No Difference

Before now, I was just growing older, and it's as simple as that. I could tell I was getting older by the way my body began to look and feel with each passing year. Every year after age thirty, something small changed. Come on Ladies, some of you over thirty know what I'm talking about. Those subtle changes like breasts not as perky and a little more jiggle on the legs, thighs, tummy, and hips. How about the heartburn after eating what you used to eat with no problem or needing a little more sleep to function properly the next day? Please don't forget about getting a little more winded at times or not moving as fast in general. All of this seems to begin in our 30s and continues to haunt us indefinitely as we grow older.

What I can attest to is that running has changed 90% of all of these "aging ailments" for me. My breasts are not as droopy and my legs don't have as much jiggle anymore. This is just a sample of how running can help you age gracefully. I know…for some of you in your 30s, 40s, and way beyond, this is the best news since sliced bread! Previously, I have provided you with examples on how running will help you physically, emotionally, mentally, and spiritually…NOW you know it can be your own little fountain of youth. How awesome is that?!!!

Seeing Your Transformation

As women, our bodies are absolutely amazing! Our bodies have the ability to do so much when we put it to the test. As women, the best thing we can do for ourselves is embrace our beautiful bodies! Once we embrace our bodies and accept our bodies, we can then appreciate the transformation that will take place as a result of running.

With every fitness goal you conquer, you will see your body transforming. Some of the transformations you will notice right away, other phases of the transformation will come later, but don't let this be discouraging. You may actually feel the difference before you see a difference. For example, you will notice very early on within the first 3 to 6 months, that you will have more strength, endurance, and more energy throughout the day. You will also be less winded, more focused, alert, and less irritable. Your energy level by this time will begin to be off the charts! We have so much more energy from running. It's amazing how we feel after our runs. You, too, will begin to have those same wonderful feelings. If you are not feeling energized, you may not be getting enough rest. Make sure if you can get your 7-8 hours of sleep.

If you are running to lose weight you may begin to drop weight within the 3 to 6-month timeframe as well. However, if you are running for a lifestyle change, you may notice around the 6 month to 12-month mark that you are more toned all over, and not just in those 'problem areas.'

Running is slimming and that's just another awesome benefit! In either case, be patient. Becoming a runner is a lifestyle change and eventually your body will follow. It has no other choice. There are so many internal, as well as external, trans-formations that take place so just stay with it, and we promise you will reap all these fabulous benefits.

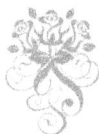

TIP

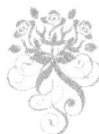

Running can give you a perfect combination
of enhancing yourself physically, mentally, and spiritually…that is simply "Smelling the Roses!"

Yolanda "Smelling the Roses" on Seeing Your Transformation

Finally, the fun part begins!!! Honestly for me the sight of the first transformation that I saw for myself, took a year for me to see. I think I was just so focused on my routine that by the time I noticed, a year was approaching. People who knew me saw changes in my body within 3–6 months. It really started with my face and neck. It seems others will notice your transfor-mation before you begin to see the changes.

At the one-year mark, I was nowhere near where I wanted to be, only to the point where it was slightly noticeable to me, but very noticeable to others. Although I was not where I wanted to be physically, mentally I had accomplished making running a consistent part of my life and that was success to me! That was still very motivating for me. It made me say, "I can't wait to see where I am in the next 6 months." Well, not only did that next 6 months come around quickly, but the two-year mark did also.

At the two-year mark, I recall feeling that my face, neck, and stomach were all a little smaller. I also recall saying, "If I had not started this walking and/or running, what would I look like now."

I was mentally happy with the thought of, "if this leads to me not ever gaining and just maintaining my weight, I am okay with that!" But, that is not what happened. By the beginning of the third year, I started getting so many compliments from many who knew the old me. I had finally arrived. Just about every day I stop and think of how I never gave up and just stayed consistent.

After three years, I really did not focus on how I looked. I just knew how good I was feeling. I can't wait for you to experience that feeling, too.

Yolanda (Before & After)

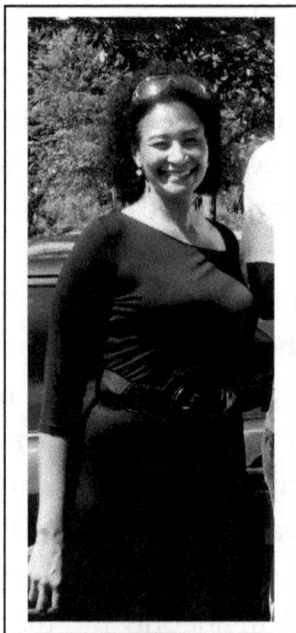

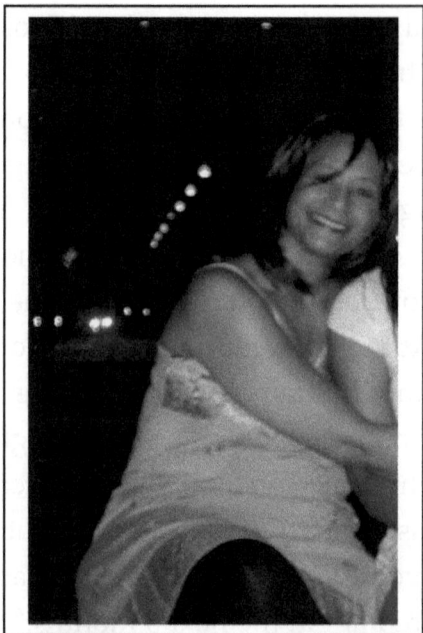

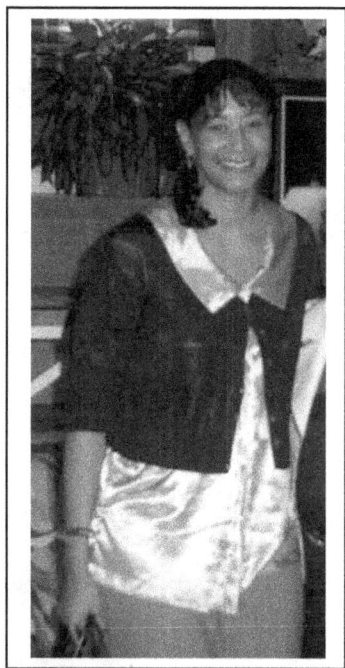

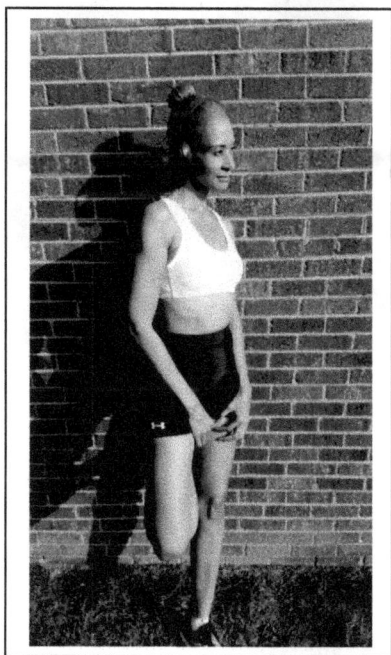

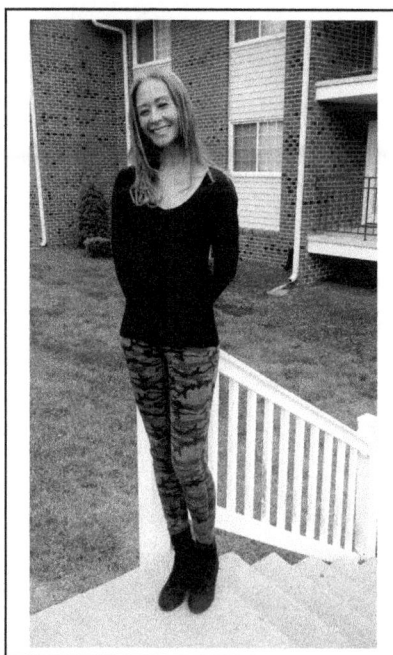

Yolanda Diaz and Itarsha Payne

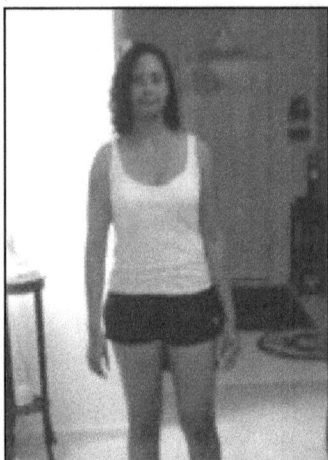

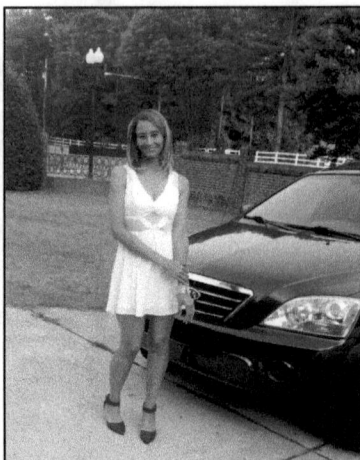

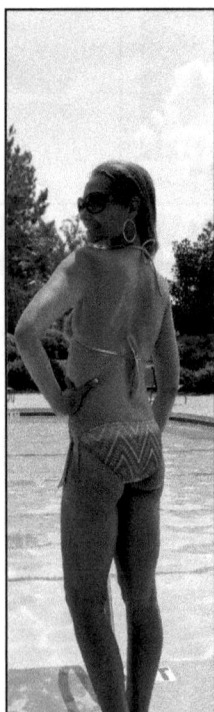

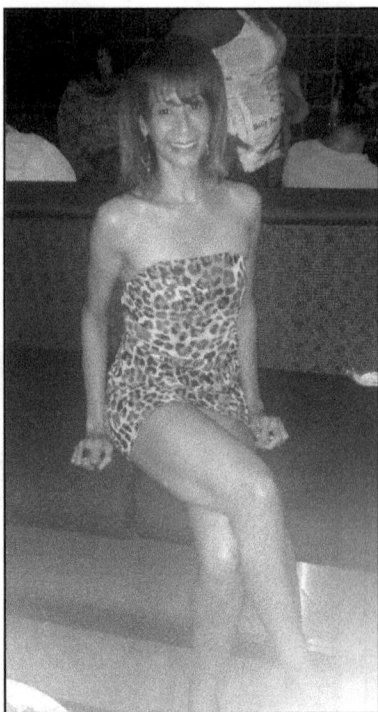

Itarsha "Smelling the Roses" on Seeing Your Transformation

Let me just say for me, there were many stages of transformation. Some came sooner rather than later. Some were physically noticeable and others weren't. The first thing I noticed was the change in my attitude towards running. Like what was mentioned earlier on: becoming a runner wasn't planned. When I began running, things became clearer and I was more focused. I felt less stressed, and I must say, I even felt happier. I just became a better version of me. Those feelings are what still make me look forward to running today.

Physically, I have noticed dramatic changes in my body. Not necessarily a drop in weight, but it looked just more toned and lean. By no means am I "skinny" or do I desire to be. It's just that I, like many other woman, noticed that my skin began to lose elasticity throughout the years and there were "things" that took a total different shape than when I was in my twenties. What I notice now is that my legs are toned, my waist seems smaller, and even my arms and back are toned. I haven't dropped actual "weight" in years. I still weigh the same and just after 5 or 6 years went down one more size. It's just that I can tell that with consistency, my body will continue to change, and it's at a pace that I am truly comfortable with, as I continue to run to be healthier.

I still feel like me but better. I feel strong, confident, positive, focused, and happier. For me the internal transformation far outweighs the external. It's weird because everyone notices the outer transformations more than I do. I guess since it's a lifestyle change and I run for the enjoyment of it, I don't really see what others see.

I want you to focus on how you feel more than what you look like. You have to remember that your body WILL change throughout your journey of becoming a runner, as long as you stay committed and consistent. So pay attention to your internal changes, because the way you feel will be what keeps you going.

Itarsha (Before & After)

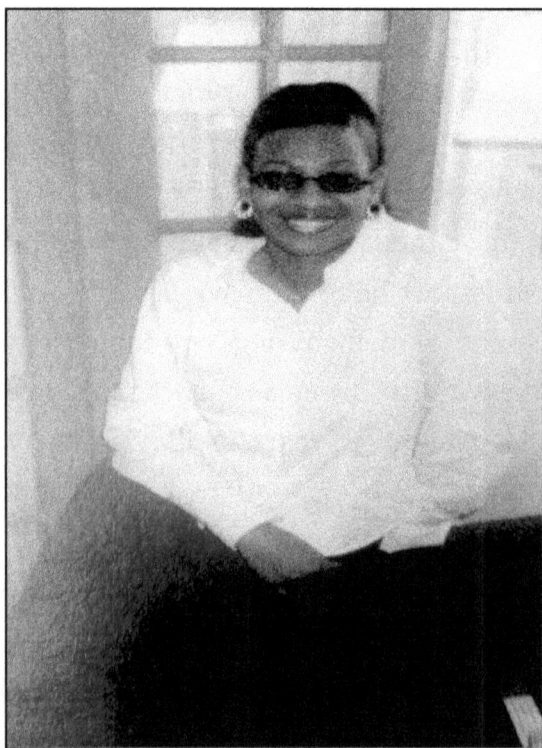

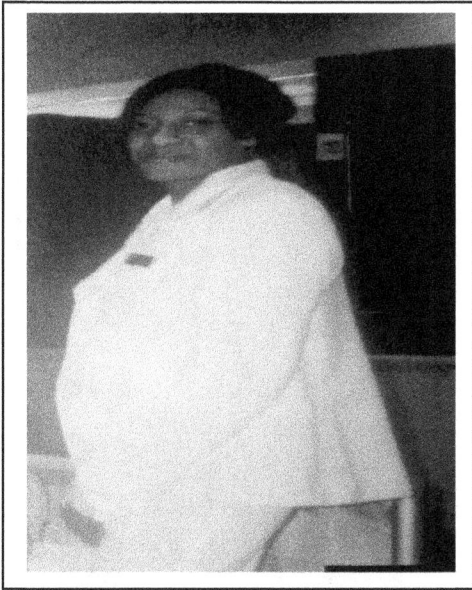
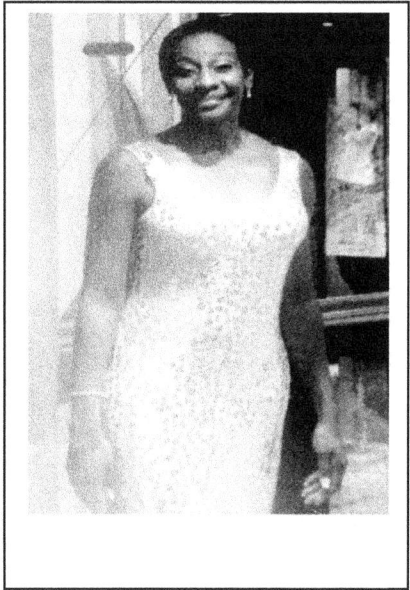
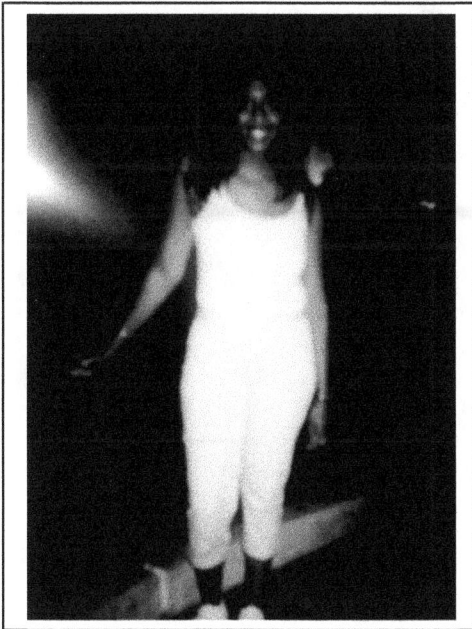
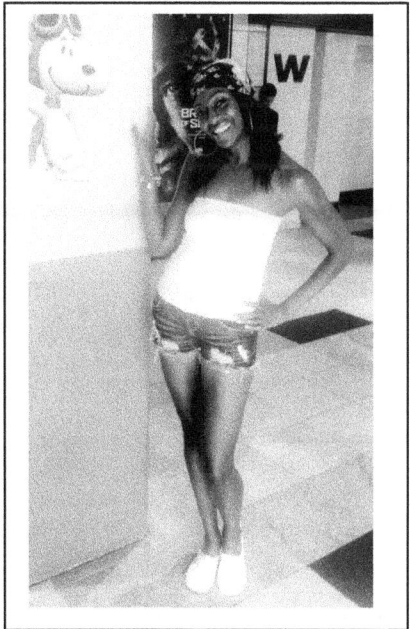

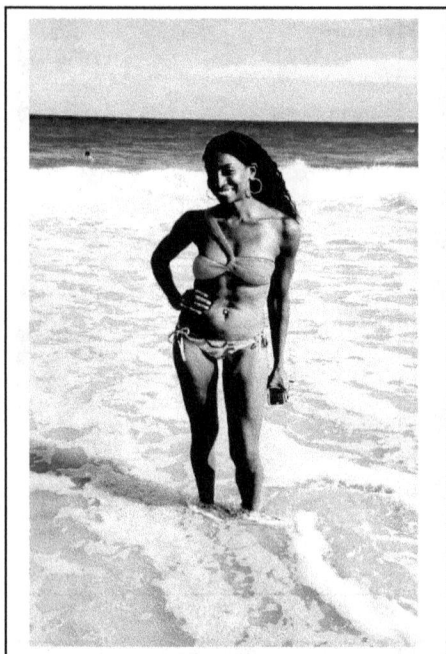
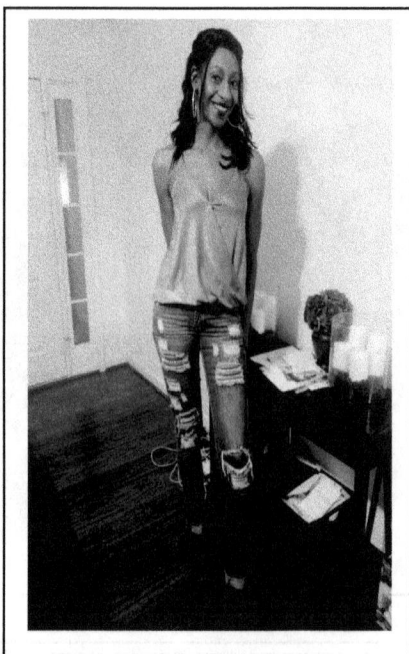
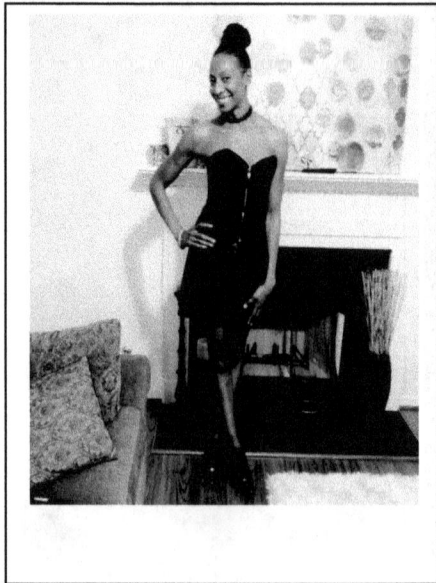
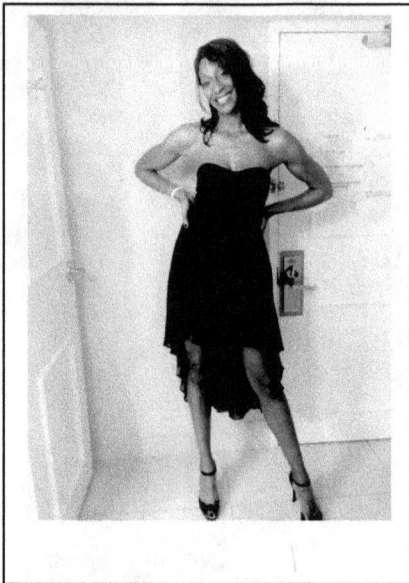

When The Unexpected Happens

We have all been down the path of dealing with an unexpected situation, circumstance, or just plain STRESS that can sometimes come down the pipe all at once. This is a part of life we all have to deal with at some point. Boy-o-boy do we know about the unexpected!

One or several things in your life can change in the blink of an eye, which can then cause a ripple effect in other areas of your life. We both have had a few life altering occurrences in the past years throughout our journey. Based on what is going on in your life, stressful events are just going to happen. We are not talking about stressful events related to running. We are talking about everyday life stress. You know what we are talking about: up all night with a sick child, you're sick, a break up, a family disagreement, etc.

We can't count the number of stressful situations we have encountered during this journey. Our bodies all react to stress in different ways—some don't eat, some eat too much, some don't sleep, etc. It can be mentally exhausting. We both have experienced divorce and other stressful situations and some mornings based on what happened the day before, with God's grace we were able to get up and stay committed to our journey. One or both of us have encountered illness, injury, divorce, financial issues, a family or friend in need—you name it, one or both of us have experienced it! Why do these things seem to happen when things are going great? Well that's because it's called "life."

Even some of the much less serious smaller unexpected things, such as a flat tire, forgetting your iPod (OMG running with no music!!), or any other little thing that can affect your run, throw you off, or turn you off from wanting to run that day, can suck big time!

We have had to push through these situations and circumstances and continue on our journey. Just think, if we had stopped running when the unexpected happened, it wouldn't help the situation or change the circumstances. So continuing on our journey for the most part keeps one thing in our life constant and normal at an uncertain time. We want to encourage you to do the same. You will feel so much better that you are continuing to take care of "you" at a time of adversity. You will actually feel stronger as a woman for it. Here you are having to deal with something outside of your control and at the same time continue to stay on track with something important to you and your health. It's a great feeling!

Just remember, it's not what happens in life; it's how you respond to it. Will you give up? Give in? Lose faith? Sometimes you may, but as long as you get up, brush yourself off and keep your mind on the commitment you made to yourself, you can weather any storm. Like we said, we definitely have weathered a few storms, and still do. We have come to realize at our age that things like this are just a part of life. The unexpected comes with living life and it's inevitable. However, you must always remember that "this too shall pass." Trust us, it will!

We have been through all of the situations listed above and through the grace of God; we have always found a way to not let it affect our journey. I truly believe it is a way for God to show you how resilient you are; otherwise, you would not know.

When we respond to the unexpected in a calm, positive way, it allows us to think more clearly about the best plan to put into action. We do this every day for our employer, when the unexpected happens on the job. And, we still get the job done.

Don't let an unexpected situation throw you off your course. You must and will find a way to get through it. Pray and reach out for support from your circle. If necessary, reevaluate your running schedule and try your best to come up with an alternate plan to stay on track to your commitment. Let your test in life be your testimony to others. It is so true when we take the first step, God will take the next. Through God and commitment, all things are possible even when the unexpected happens.

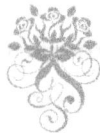

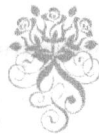

TIP
Keep a spare gym bag
with all of your running gear in your car at all times, so you will always be prepared if the unexpected happens.

Itarsha "Smelling the Roses" on When The Unexpected Happens...

Wow! Let's see, where do I begin? In June 2012, I cracked my hip unbeknownst to me. I'm not really sure how I did it, but for three months, I walked around thinking I had a pulled groin injury that would eventually heal. I went back and forth to the doctor and a regular X-ray didn't show anything, so my doctor continued to chalk it up to a slow healing groin pull. I was in severe pain every day for three months and unable to run because of the constant pain. I was in so much pain I asked for a steroid shot, walked on a cane, took off work to rest, but nothing was helping. Over a three-month period, the pain just got progressively worse. My equilibrium was off, so I kept tripping and falling, on top of being in so much pain. My doctor finally felt the need to order an MRI. The day after the MRI was performed, I fell one last time and completely broke my hip. That was September 9, 2012.

After emergency surgery and a hospital stay, I ended up with a plate and 3 pins in my left hip. For a total of six months, from June 2012 thru December 2012, I was consumed with severe pain every day. At any point during that six-month period, I had hip surgery, physical therapy, was in a wheelchair, on a walker, had to use crutches, restricted to bed rest and also had to use a cane. I really thought running, even walking correctly without assistance, was a thing of the past. This took a huge toll on me, not only physically, but mentally, emotionally, and spiritually. I was deeply saddened.

Today, through the grace of God, I am 100% recovered and healed! I actually run faster and further, and I'm more fit and happier than I've ever been. God puts no more on us than we can handle. I'm a testimony that **GOD IS REAL** and through prayer and faith in His Word, He will see you through anything. I give God all the praise, glory, and honor!

Was it a tough journey? Absolutely! Very much so! The hardest thing I have ever gone through and had to overcome in my entire life, **physically, mentally, and emotionally**. If it were not for God, then I wouldn't have been sustained. With God's help, I used every ounce of determination, dedication, and commitment to myself and Yolanda to rehabilitate myself. The worst part is that I had to go it alone, because I couldn't or wouldn't think of trying to hinder Yolanda's progress. I've shared this to show you that your test can be your testimony, and it must not deter you from what God has for you. He wants us all to be happy and live wonderful, healthy lives. It's up to us to follow his plan. So ladies, when the unexpected happens, you must lean on God and dig deep inside and find that determination to adapt. Trust me, it's there, and you can find it. Trust God. If I did it, you can, too!

Yolanda "Smelling the Roses" on When The Unexpected Happens...

My, my, my you name it, I had it — stress in all shapes and sizes. Sometimes the night before I ran, some type of adversity would appear for me to deal with and I would say, "There is no way I am going to be able to get up and run." Somehow God just makes my determination to get up and run happen. I get up, I get out, and I start running. I truly believe running while you are under stress, is the best remedy for stress. I always feel much better about the situation and have more clarity about what direction I should take in a calmer and peaceful way. It is very difficult running and wanting to cry about something at the same time. You just want to give up and stop, but as you go a little further, you realize how your body just wants to keep going and you let it. That to me is God's way of showing us how strong we are and can be.

When something is working well, you naturally learn to stick to it and expect it to always work well. For many reasons, you may be forced to change what you are used to. There will come a time when the unexpected happens. When Itarsha injured her hip, the unexpected incident forced me to have to change my entire way of thinking, my routine, and much more. I did not realize how much I relied on her being there. I had to get up each morning and rely on myself for motivation! I did it and you can, too! I had to change to a routine that worked best for me, since I was running alone. It is amazing what you can do when you never give up!

In 2015, I was rear ended in a car accident by a car going 50 mph. I had a rotator cuff injury and a hip/back injury in addition to a mild concussion and a few other injuries. I had a specialist for every injury. I was so upset and thought I may not be able to run the same again. When I told my orthopedic doctor I was a runner, he told me that I can heal with the proper physical therapy for my shoulder, hip, back, and neck to avoid surgery. I could not run for six months, but I made sure I did what the doctors told me, and I went to therapy so that I could get better. I listened to what each doctor told me to do for my injuries. It takes time when your body is older, and it does not bounce back like it does in our 20's or 30's. It is devastating to be a runner and not be able to run. After six months, I was running, but nowhere near the speed and pace that I had worked up to before the accident. It took me eight months to get back to that level. I learned so much about my body due to my injuries, such as how to heal it with proper treatment. Unfortunately, due to the accident, I will never be 100% without aches and pains at times, but I know how to comfort the pain, because I gained information about how I should proceed after the accident as a runner. I am so glad to have avoided surgery. There are many unexpected things that can and will happen. You just got to develop a plan B and sometimes C. Some of the unexpected events that may happen to you will be an incident that at first seems like a major issue. Once you take time to think of a strategy, sometimes the issue ends up teaching you that you are stronger than you ever knew. I found this out by learning to run alone at times, due to Itarsha's hip tragedy and also with the accident I was in that gave me injuries. We both learned how strong we were and we were able to come back stronger and faster than ever.

Chapter 8

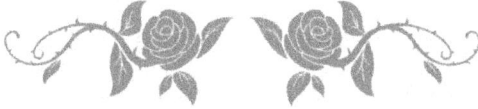

DON'T "HATE" TILL YOU KNOW WHAT IT TAKES

W hen you first read the title to this chapter, you may be unaware of what we mean and what we are saying. We promise you at some point after you have been in your running routine for six months or more, you will refer back to this chapter and relate to it 100%.

When your body begins to transform, **GET READY! THE HATERS** will begin their attack. We are in no way negative people, but this is reality. Here are some examples of what you might experience:

- They will try and schedule something with you when they know darn well that is the time you are committed to running!
- They will say "don't get too skinny" and what you are doing is going to make you "too skinny!"
- They will cook you pies and cakes and try to get you to eat lots of all the wrong things. And don't forget there are always cookies and cupcakes in the break room at work!
- Many outings will include food, food, and more FOOD!

Some people say everyday "I want to do this" or "I want to be this way," but they are not willing to put the work in for any of their desires, so they hate on your desires to be healthy. **BUT YOU** have made the decision to **Do What It Takes for You** and for that you should commend yourself!

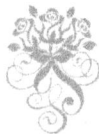

TIP

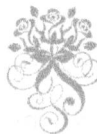

Never accept what other people perceive as YOUR limitations when it comes to running.

If your body allows you to run, then there is no reason you can't run.

Yolanda "Smelling the Roses" on Don't Hate Till You Know What It Takes!

Congratulations! The healthy body that God blessed you with has arrived. You did it! No surgery and no pills! You will be so amazed at how your body has changed! The good news is that not only has your body changed, but your mind and spirit as well! Now that is some serious balance and you really do need all three: Mind, Body, and Soul! Here comes the fun part! Getting dressed to go somewhere has never been this fun or easy! But, dealing with the reaction of your new look from others has never been harder! I started with a lot of weight on me and Itarsha was transforming way before me. She was my motivation. I have a very easygoing personality and just love all people. Honestly, she warned me about how I would be treated by some people while my body is changing. I never thought I would see it, but she was right.

You, like I, will experience first-hand the looks of hateration from strangers and people you least expect. It can make you feel very uncomfortable and hurt. You may not realize it is even happening. Just be aware! You have changed right before people's eyes. There will be compliments and there will be statements that will embarrass you and seem insulting. Here are some of the following comments I heard:

- Where did your big butt go?
- Where did your stomach go?
- Girl you need to put some meat on those bones.
- I liked you better when you were bigger.

It's something that you will have to adjust to, but never let it get you down. You worked hard for what you have, so be proud no matter what!

Itarsha "Smelling the Roses" on Don't Hate Till You Know What It Takes!

I have a very interesting story: My ex-husband and I spent several holidays with his family when we were married. On this particular year, we were spending Thanksgiving at his mother's house. Since we live in North Carolina, and most of his family lives in Florida, we didn't see or spend time with them often throughout the year. When I got married in 2002 I had dieted and exercised down to a size 10 for my wedding day and stayed that size for years, until I began my journey. His family would see me year after year, and I was pretty much the same size, until this particular year. I think when I went from a size 10 to a size 8 it was a huge difference in the way I looked because not only did I lose weight, I lost inches and my body was toning all over making me look even smaller. So what happened on this particular Thanksgiving? I caught a family member staring at me and my big plate of food, that's what happened! It was odd and uncomfortable. This person couldn't take their eyes off me and my plate.

Ladies, when I'm not watching what I eat, I'm REALLY NOT watching what I eat! I get my eat on! The look on this person's face said, "I bet she isn't going to eat all of that." Her thoughts seemed to be transparent. I can tell she may have felt I was too "small" and surely got that way by not eating.

That occurrence along with comments from people in general gave me a complex. Can you believe that I have a complex about being sizes smaller than people were used to seeing me? I have a complex about being "thin."

I'm naturally an optimistic person. I know people have problems with accepting change, good or bad, but good change should come with positive support and encouragement from others. However, in the real world, that's not always the case. So I guess what I'm trying to say is don't be surprised if your family, friends, and co-workers don't celebrate you as much as you think they should for your new body, because it will take time for them to warm up to the new you.

Don't take it too personal. And, please don't let it stop you. You are doing what makes YOU happy and that's what matters. Whether you are happy with being a size 16 or a size 6, or that you came down from a size 26 or a size 16, you did it! So be proud!

Getting up to run three days a week is no easy feat. It's hard work, and I just think all hard work deserves compensation. My compensation for my hard work is a healthier me. The awesome thing about living a healthier lifestyle is that anyone can do it. My goal is to help anyone that wishes to run-for-their-life to do so. Ladies, let the haters hate, while you and I do what it takes!

Strength Training

We believe that some form of strength or endurance training should be part of any fitness regimen. A body shouldn't survive on cardio alone. Strength training helps keep your muscles and bones strong, and that's a very good thing! As we mentioned previously, we run every other day approximately three days a week. We do strength/endurance training two to three days a week, on the days we do not run. Strength training is a very important part of being fit. We feel that it helps our running as well. We suggest you research and see what type of strength or endurance training is good for you. Doing your own research will help you customize what is best for your body type.

Yolanda "Smelling the Roses" on Strength Training

Strength training is a nice change from running. I do not lift very heavy weights. I need to tone up flab and consistent strength training will do just that. You also get a wonderful release of endorphins that make you feel great after strength training. You want your body to have some form of definition, and it truly makes a difference. I love it!

Itarsha "Smelling the Roses" on Strength Training

I have to admit that I didn't begin strength training to become stronger or more toned. I originally began strength training to "not look skinny." I'm really tall, and I have to be careful about

142

losing weight because I can end up looking like a stick pole! That to me is not attractive, so I incorporated strength training into my regimen. I don't lift heavy weights. I am not radical with it either. Just a few times a week keeps me toned and shapely without have that "skinny" look.

Ladies, don't be afraid to pick up light weights a few times a week. Strength training will tone out your beautiful runner's body!

Don't Give Up

We know by this time you are saying to yourself, "How am I going to do this? There is so much more to running than I knew." We say to you in return, "Take it one run at a time." As we explained to you earlier, we didn't wake up one morning, put on our gear, and hit the streets. It was a very gradual trans-formation, as it will be for you. Most importantly is whatever you do, DON'T GIVE UP! It took several months through trial and error for us to get it right, and we are still learning different things in terms of running, shoes, clothing, etc. It's truly a journey that we are blessed to be able to take and enjoy. However, we, too, get tired and discouraged. Sometimes, we have to dig deep inside to push out that one last mile, or even one last step! Many times after a run, we will head inside to get ready for work and still be amazed as to how we did it!

We'd think: *It is 22 degrees today and we ran five miles outside in the freezing cold!* We often think the next time it will not be possible. However, when the time comes, we find ourselves doing it one more time. This is what you truly call "one-run-at-a-time" in action.

We all desire to accomplish goals in life, but sometimes we have a hard time focusing long enough to stay committed to fulfilling that goal. We all have fallen short in some areas of our lives when we have called it quits. We said all that to say: We know you will feel tired, discouraged, mentally, and physically drained because we do at times. However, always remember, that anything worth having is worth working for and doesn't come without hard work and determination. So whether it's a healthier you, a thinner you, or both, DON'T GIVE UP!

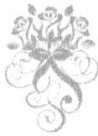

TIP

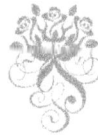

Fear can keep you from
reaching your running potential. Fear of failing or worrying about
what others think can hinder you. You must release the fear and have
faith.

Itarsha "Smelling the Roses" on Don't Give Up!

Don't give up, hang in there! I know it's easier said than done; however, the payoff is huge. When I was growing up, I used to watch people do what they love in amazement. Politicians,

Olympic athletes, workaholics, and anyone that I knew or saw giving 110% always wowed me. I never felt that way before about anything, except raising my son, but that was natural as a mother. I'm talking about that feeling of loving to do something when it's on my mind all the time, or being excited about the next time I'm going to do it. Enjoying every minute and making sure other things are scheduled around it. I've found that joy in running and I feel blessed because of it. It feels good to be passionate about something that's positive and contributes to a healthier me. It also feels good to be a catalyst in helping you reach your fitness goals through my journey. So giving up is not a desire for me because the benefits are just too awesome! Yes, the feeling comes, but easy come, easy go...that's my motto when it comes to giving up on running or giving up on you!

Ladies, I want to share this feeling with you. I want to help you not give up. You may not get the same satisfaction as I do out of running, but you WILL GET the same benefits. I want you to experience the benefits. So dig deep and don't give up because you are worth it and so much more.

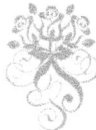

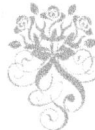

TIP
Running gives you a taste of life
on a whole new level and can teach you so much about yourself.

Yolanda Diaz and Itarsha Payne

Yolanda "Smelling the Roses" on Don't Give Up!

Don't give up! These three words we hear and will continue to hear many, many times throughout our life. This is what was told to us as children, and this is what we tell our children. As soon as I heard these words, I honestly would feel the weight of the goal I wanted to accomplish come over me. It seemed like a dark cloud. When and if that happens to you, have your source of positive power ready to go and to zap yourself with it.

Your source of power can be many things: a moment in prayer, a sample picture of the body you are designing, or calling a friend. Take time to write a list of your sources of power. This list will truly come in handy. Just take it one day at a time, one week, one month, or even one year at a time. Something is driving me and I truly feel it is several power sources. One power source that really drives me is the statistics of obesity and heart disease for Hispanics and African Americans and being a role model for others, so I can help them. Something will make you get up, get out, and do it!

Each day, you get closer and closer to your goals and before you know it, it is one year later. Stay on track and visualize your end results every day.

At times, I did not know where the motivation came from, and then I realized that God is powerful and I must give him praise and thanks. I would have never succeeded without Him. Thank you God for helping me to NEVER give up!

Chapter 9

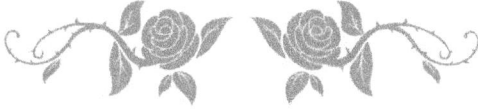

REST AND RELAXATION

Please understand that as we share our journey, we want you to realize that it's so very important to get the proper rest and relaxation. You have worked hard and each week, you need to be sure to insert time in your schedule to get rest, relax, and just enjoy YOU. We make sure we take time to do this. Your form of relaxation may be different from others, and it's not just about lying down. It could be a nice walk in a garden or reading a book on your back porch. Your form of relaxation does not have to be alone time. It could be going to the park with your kids or going to get an ice cream treat. Rest and relaxation go hand and hand.

Some people cannot go to bed as early as others. We are also referring to some vacation time, a week or a weekend out of town. Your mind, body, and soul will get rejuvenated and become more strengthened for your next run.

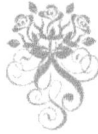

TIP

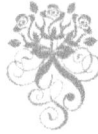

Take at least two annual short breaks
from running to allow yourself time to rejuvenate. Don't be afraid of losing fitness gains, when you return back to running, you will be stronger and more focused.

Yolanda "Smelling the Roses" on Rest And Relaxation

I cannot tell you how exciting it is to decide what my weekly R&R (Rest and Relaxation) is going to consist of for myself. There are so many things that come to my mind. They are mostly based on the weather. If it is too cold for me to go outside, it may be a day of watching movies and eating my favorite popcorn.

For some reason, most of my relaxation involves eating a nice meal or snack. If it is a nice day, I am happy reading on my back porch or having family and/or friends over for a "bring your own dish" cookout. The food, the laughter, and the rest are all so very therapeutic to me and very necessary.

In addition, to your favorite R&R activity, it is so very important to get the proper rest. If you do not get enough sleep, it can affect your run. I try to get as much rest as I can. Yes, I have to skip my favorite TV shows that come on after 9PM, and I do.

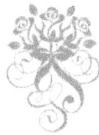

TIP

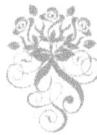

After a run, *don't rush right back into life. Take a few minutes to walk, stretch or meditate.*

Itarsha "Smelling the Roses" on Rest and Relaxation

When running I am fully engaged, because I simply love to run. However, when it's time to rest, I'm so ready for it and look forward to my time of R&R. I primarily run during the week and rest on the weekends. So Friday is almost like Christmas Eve sometimes! I can't wait to lounge around the house, watch movies, and snack on Saturday morning. When it's nice out, I like to sit by the pool and read or write.

Mostly, anything that is not physical is rest for me. I appreciate my rest time, because I know my body, mind, and spirit needs the rest, as well as craves it. Once that need and craving is satisfied, then my body will reward me by becoming better and stronger. Yours will, too, when you give your body the rest it needs.

Keep A Photographic Journal

Pictures are truly worth a thousand words! So ladies snap, snap, snap away! When you begin your journey find that before picture, because your picture one month later, three months later, six months later and a one year later picture will all reflect different stages and tell your fantastic story.

Take all kinds of pictures: right, left, front, back, and even naked (for you and your significant other...lol) before, during, and after you've reached your fitness goals. Just remember being fit is a lifetime commitment that never ends, so never stop snapping!

We have probably taken more pictures throughout our journey than we've taken in our lives. So trust us ladies, you'll get really good at taking pictures!

Yolanda "Smelling the Roses" on Keeping A Photographic Journal

I am so happy I have pictures to help and show people to see where I have been and where I am now. These before and after pictures keep me motivated. I don't know what I would do without them. I, like others, had the moment when I saw myself in "**THAT**" picture, prior to being on my journey that made me say, "**OH MY GOODNESS**" I have got to get this under control. Don't ever let time go by where it has been more than three months when you do not have photos. Photos are your motivation at all times; at the beginning and during your lifestyle change.

Itarsha "Smelling the Roses" on Keeping A Photographic Journal

The first thing I want to say about taking pictures is: They do not lie! Pictures tell the raw truth—be it good or bad. When a picture is bad, it's really bad! I have pictures from years ago that don't even look like me. I have literally shown pictures to people and they've said "Who is this?" They are somewhat shocked when I reveal that it's me in the picture. My transformation has not only transformed my body, but also my face. I look older ten years ago in some pictures than my current age. Now that I have reached my fitness goals, I continue to take pictures to keep myself on track.

Yes, I can look in the mirror to see changes in my body. However, there is something about "a moment in time;" pictures capture the truth of that moment. The good news is these pictures keep me motivated to continue on my journey, simply because I love how I look in the mirror and in pictures. And, it's a wonderful feeling. Don't worry, you will get to this point. So ladies, keep transforming those bodies and keep snapping those pictures and watch yourself reach your fitness goals.

Becoming A Role Model

At first glance, what do you think about when you see those two words in the chapter's header? Most people don't think of fitness gurus or personal trainers. What about regular individuals that are trying to live a healthier lifestyle and to live a longer more fulfilling life? Nope, most people don't think of them as role models either, but guess what? We do, we think they are! So we are here to hopefully be role models to you, and in return, we hope you pay-it-forward to your family and friends.

Let's talk about the fitness industry for a minute. Right off the top of your head, can you think of any minority women in the fitness industry? There is only one that comes to mind without actual research. We have all heard of her. She's a certain celebrity's ex-wife. Other than that, it will take a little bit of research to find some others. The other thing is, although they may be out there, they are not prominent and we should put some of the blame on "us."

You ask why we partially blame "us?" Well for starters, fitness professionals are not in great demand in our community. Some of you may not like what we're saying, but we are speaking the truth. Society operates on supply and demand. The more society wants then the more society gets. If minority communities are not making demands on the fitness industry by educating ourselves and our families on the importance of fitness, and also pushing for more facilities, parks, and even sidewalks in our neighborhoods, things will not change.

The further into our journey we ventured, the more we realized the above. Once our love of running and a healthier lifestyle began to "catch on" for our friends, family, and co-workers, they began to look to us for tips on what we are doing to get in shape and stay in shape. We now constantly hear from them and even from strangers about how great we look. People come up to both of us and ask, "What are you doing to stay in shape?" We simply answer, "We run." We both hope to one day become role models to women everywhere. We want to help raise awareness in our community of the importance of fitness.

Family needs to help family first. At our traditional family reunions, we usually sit around eating the pig, the fried chicken, mac-n-cheese, cornbread, macaroni salad, and BBQ ribs, and we won't even go into the desserts! Let's change the game, ladies. Why not schedule a 3K walk or run in the itinerary one morning during the reunion? We need to start thinking outside the box and begin incorporating some physical activities into our gatherings. Doing so will make everyone feel better, and who knows, it may be the beginning of a "Smelling the Roses" moment for some.

It is always so rewarding when you can help and inspire others with your experiences. We want this book not only to motivate those who want to run, but to also motivate someone to step up, take the lead, and say, "I need to help my friend or loved one, and I need to commit to helping them today and be the support they need."

If you are the fit one, help someone else and GET UP! Helping others isn't about you, it's about them. But, guess what?

Your commitment to helping them live a healthier lifestyle, keeps you motivated to continue on your journey of becoming even stronger as a role model to someone else. So at the end of the day, you ARE helping yourself and EVERYONE WINS!

Yolanda "Smelling the Roses" on Becoming A Role Model

Deep down inside of us, we all have the desire to want to help others. For me, I have had this desire since my childhood. Helping others has always been a calling of mine. We have all had that thought...hmmm? I wish I could do this or that for someone. Well, being a role model for my family was the best thing I felt I could do for them and others. When I look back to when I was about eleven or so, I remember my mother working out all the time. Now that I am 49 and I look back, she was a great role model for me, but at that time, I did not realize it.

Today, my mother has inspired me with her physically fit body at the age of 68. When I was at my heaviest weight, seeing her would remind me of what the body I know God gave me should somewhat look like. Please don't misunderstand me when I talk about my body when I was bigger. I still was happy with who I was and loved the accomplishments I had made in my life with my daughter and my career, but I found an even happier me that I did not know existed when I dropped the extra weight.

Once you accomplish bringing out the real body God has designed for you, being a role model to help others to do the same will be so very rewarding. You are actually contributing by physically, mentally, and spiritually saving lives!

In the beginning, I was just looking to be more fit and healthier, and I never imagined I would be more mentally transformed than physically. For me the mental transformation is actually worth more than the physical. Love who you are and who you are becoming every step of the way. No matter what your body size is, as long as you are doing what you can do to be fit, you are winning!

Itarsha "Smelling the Roses" on Becoming A Role Model

Role model? Who me? The tall shy girl that never spoke or approached anyone first in high school. I could never see myself as a role model and really still don't. Many of my friends tell me that I am an inspiration to them. I have even had strangers ask me what I do. Early mornings when I am running, I see some of the same cars drive by and some of the people wave as they pass me by. I also notice people are walking more in my neighborhood.

The meaning of "role model" has certainly changed for me now that I'm a runner. Before now, I looked at a role model as someone who makes a huge impact in the lives of many people all at once. Someone who has notoriety in the public eye. Someone who has caused a major positive ripple effect that will impact society in a huge way. Little did I know how wrong I had been.

I now know a role model can have a positive effect on one person in a very small way and it still can have a HUGE impact in their life. It feels good to be an inspiration and encourage others through my hard work, discipline, and dedication to running. God's plan is for me to inspire others and that's why he blessed me with the determination to keep going, and to "show" others that anyone can be a role model and encourage others in a positive way. Who knew?

Enjoy Your New Cheerleaders

Well we warned you about the "haters," but in the end you will have more fans than haters and your own fan club! In addition to your family members and your new fan club members, there will be people you would never suspect. You will be quite surprised by the strangers who will just walk up to you and let you know you are looking great! It can be your grocery store clerks and people who see you in your day-to-day life. Even where you normally go for lunch, someone who works there will compliment you.

As you run down the street, you will recognize cars that are truly giving a supported honk and thumbs up out of the window. You will even have strangers roll down their window and pull up next to you and say, "Good for you. I need to be out there, too."

When we started our journey, we did not see people that look like us running in our neighborhood. After approximately six months or so, we began to see a few women walking and some even jogging. Sometimes, without being acknowledged, you will inspire others — that to us is such a good feeling!

Itarsha "Smelling the Roses" on Enjoy Your New Cheerleaders

What's funny about having a "new fan club" is that some of them are the same people that used to hate on me or throw shade my way at the beginning of my journey. Now I get compliments from the majority of them, along with others.

I attend a local gym and many of the "regulars" see me often, but still come up to me and give me a thumbs up or an encouraging word. It's nice to know that others are being inspired by my hard work. People in stores and public places come up and ask me what I do and tell me that I look great. One compliment that I ABSOLUTELY love is when people guess my age to be in the 30's! Come on ladies admit it, all of us love this! I guess what I'm saying is that self -motivation is great and will ultimately be what keeps you on track with your journey. However, encouraging words and accolades from others is a great motivator, too!

Yolanda "Smelling the Roses" on Enjoy Your New Cheerleaders

Realizing there are people who are truly sincere and motivating was an unexpected benefit to the rewards of my accomplishment. It took a while for it to sink in. When I first started getting compliments, I was in shock. Oh my goodness, they were saying this to me! At times, I would run into a very loud fan of my weight loss, and they would say very loudly some of the following comments: "Girl, where did the other half of you go?" or "I remember you, you were much, much bigger!" I knew at the end of the day, they meant well, and I appreciated it. It is always nice to be reminded where you came from.

The most rewarding compliments I get come from young girls in high school or women not more than twenty-five. For example, they would say, "Oh my goodness I want to be fit like you. What do you do?" I have had young girls ask if they can run with me. They are reaching out to me for help and I love mentoring them. One of my most frequent bits of information I give them is that you must first love yourself no matter what size you are. Everyone has beauty inside and out. Feeling and being fit amplifies that beauty.

Chapter 10

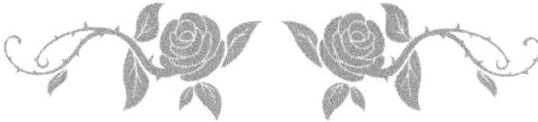

SHOPPING FOR THE NEW YOU

At the beginning of our journey, shopping wasn't on our minds. Once we began to see physical changes in our bodies, we had to make shopping a priority. "FOR GOODNESS SAKES" our original pants that we started running in, were falling down at some point! All of our clothes were becoming bigger! It's funny because we did not realize it at first. For example, we would keep tightening the belt we wore with our pants and dresses so they could fit. We finally realized we had to buy a new everything in clothes. Financially, shopping was not good, but mentally this was good and represented the results from our hard work.

Shopping for something new, as we progressed, became exciting, and something we felt was important to help keep us motivated. We needed to feel good in all the clothes we were wearing, and this meant our running gear and our day-to-day clothing. It is no fun wearing drawers and bras that are too big!

Everyone around you will begin to tell you how great you look and how you are an inspiration as they told us. What we had to realize is that we had to give ourselves "a pat on the back," too! Shopping was one of the ways we gave ourselves that pat. You can take it one step further, because it is not just about shopping for clothes. Rewarding yourself with jewelry, a new hairstyle, a massage, etc. at the end of the week or month is important. You will be feeling good and looking good! As you are on this journey stay focused on your goal and again, don't forget to reward yourself.

Itarsha "Smelling the Roses" on Shopping For the New You

Shopping! Yes! I love to shop, but prior to transforming my body to the smaller version it is now, not so much. It's already tough to shop for clothes when you are way taller than the average height woman, then try throwing in "weight" and "size" and you end up with misery!

Ladies, you know how we women like to get together to shop? Well that was never me. I would go it alone, because it used to take me FOREVER to find something or anything to fit me right. If it wasn't my 6'1" frame, it was my size 14 and expanding body. I hated trying things on to find them too short

160

and too small. Plus, everything looked weird and felt uncomfortable on my body. Currently, you ask? Well now I LOVE TO SHOP! Though I may have some of the same challenges with the length, I can now wear just about anything I want to wear, and it looks and feels great!

So I want to let those of you with the dreaded thoughts about shopping know that you, too, can fall in love with shopping. Keep doing what you're doing, because that feeling is right around the corner!

Yolanda "Smelling the Roses" on Shopping For the New You

I don't think it has really sunk in that I can go into a store and shop for the new me. I remember almost being a size 18 and trying on anything, and it became depressing. If I had five pieces of clothing to try on, the chances of any looking how I wanted them to look was hard to accomplish. A moment of acknowledgement will keep coming at you and I had to acknowledge it was not the clothes, it was me.

One of my motivations that is keeping me on this journey of smelling the roses is the joy of shopping for clothes that I now have, and it is a wonderful feeling. I worked hard to get to where I am and I work harder to stay this way. I truly can appreciate my 5'11 frame even more when shopping now. From the first three months, when we started this journey, I became excited about shopping. Make it a goal to make the "New" you arrive/or the "New" you in progress to "Get It In", shopping that is. Those new threads on that new attitude and body will have you really smelling the roses and yourself (smile)!

Go Ahead And Accept Your Compliments!

It's not a secret that most people do not know how to accept a compliment. We honestly did not know how to accept the amount of compliments and attention we received. Of course, we said, "Thank you," but we often wondered what they were seeing that we didn't. We also didn't feel that deserving of them. It's definitely something we had to work on.

At first, it will be difficult to accept compliments right away without feeling "some kind of way." You may feel uncomfortable or even embarrassed. However, over time it will become easier. We want you to be prepared and practice accepting them early on. Throughout your journey those compliments will turn into little sparks of motivation and sometimes help you through that next run, so don't turn any down!

Itarsha "Smelling the Roses" on Go Ahead and Accept Your Compliments!

For me, this was really tough. In the beginning, when I began my journey, I would get "foe" compliments, better known as "shade" thrown at me in a form of a "compliment." I guess I can say transforming into a smaller me wasn't as great to others as it was for me. As I mentioned earlier, I would hear things like, "you are going to blow away" or "you are getting TOO small!"

or I would just get strange looks when I eat, as if I'm going to do something weird or crazy with my food. So as you can probably understand, when the sincere compliments began to flow, I felt a little uncomfortable.

NOW, I not only accept my compliments, but I also feel proud when I am complimented. I have earned each and every compliment through hard work, dedication, endurance, commitment, and tenacity. I thank God every day for giving my body the capability to do what I love to do. So with my head held high and a smile on my face, I proudly say "thank you" to everyone that notices with a compliment.

Yolanda "Smelling the Roses" on Go Ahead and Accept Your Compliment!

We can't stress it enough. Get ready for the compliments and we mean the sincere compliments! From the first 10 lbs. to 50 plus lbs. they are coming to you! Don't take them for granted. You earned them.

Those compliments are like little angels cheering for you. God has his way of confirming when you are on the right road! Amen!

REFLECTIONS BEFORE AND DURING THE JOURNEY

We want you to remember that this is an ongoing journey and not a short trip. What happens on all journeys, is that you may have to continuously change course depending on the point you are at, and this is no different. Being able to look back and reflect is almost as important as the journey itself.

Reflecting helps you see your progress. You will not always notice day-to-day changes and sometimes you will only notice changes over a period of time. Taking a moment to constantly reflect weekly and monthly at each level, will give you a better understanding of who you are, and who you are becoming. Having documented our journey has allowed us to be able to reflect back to each moment during it. Your journal will allow you to reflect back to where you started and how you progressed. These reflections represent your physical, mental, and spiritual growth. You will reflect back to what you thought you could not do and could not get through, only to find you got through it. And, you did it!

Yolanda "Smelling the Roses" on Reflections

We have been through so much while on this journey, encountering stressful situations of all types. We always reflect back to the voice telling us to keep going…the voice of God. Through Him we were able to do so. Every day I have a thought of Wow!

Running over five years and thinking back to when I started, I never thought I would look and feel as good as I do at this age. Getting up 6 days a week for so many years, takes a lot of inner discipline. I just made each day about that day and I told myself tomorrow will take care of itself and the next thing I knew five years had gone by. Losing that first 10lbs was so very motivating.

The voice in my head telling me I can do it was often attached to the voice of doubt. The way I conquered it was knowing God was with me and it was not about losing weight, but it is about being healthy. The weight loss was just an extra perk in addition to many other perks. I also overcame that voice of doubt with my faith in God and myself.

You will make it to this point and you will reflect back. You will realize I can do this and anything I commit to.

Itarsha "Smelling the Roses" on Reflections

Boy has it been a journey! Yolanda and I have grown in so many ways through running and writing this book. Our friendship has become stronger, our bodies of course have become healthier and stronger, and spiritually and emotionally, we have evolved. As I write this entry, I can't help but reflect on the ups, downs, and the ins and outs I've experienced since my journey began that April in 2008. So much has changed over the years. I can't believe I've held steady to running for seven going on eight years, hardly missing a beat. It's an unbelievable, but very true testimony. Through injuries, separation and divorce, moving twice, starting two businesses full-time, encouraging and supporting my young adult son, and everything in between, I still run. God has truly sustained my body, mind, and soul through it all. Only God has allowed my body day after day, week after week, month after month, and year after year to continue to do what I love. I hope you ladies will also have the special blessing of sustaining the gift of running for years to come.

Chapter 11

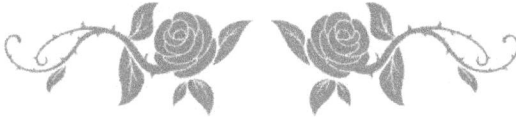

USE THE INTERNET

Free information is at your fingertips. There is so much information on the Internet to answer many questions you may have throughout your journey. The Internet is such a great resource and provides a wealth of information on fitness and running. We are also open to receiving questions and information from others that share our love for running. We will swap running tips with each other and oftentimes, they share wonderful and useful Internet resources. We are fortunate to have an abundance of information on the Internet readily available that helps runners continue to move towards doing and being their best. These resources also help keep us motivated, focused, and on track with our journey.

Don't be alarmed if you find you've been doing things wrong or could have been doing something better. We want to prevent you from making the errors we've made. However, we are still learning new things to add, take away, etc. to this day, and as time goes on, so will you.

So turning to the Internet from time to time has been our "quick fix" for something not serious enough to reach out to a professional for on our journey. We want to continue to pay-it-forward and share little tips we've found along the way on the Internet throughout the years. Don't forget to visit our website at **www.runandsmelltheroses.com** for these fantastic tips!

We Are So Proud Of You

We are so proud of you, as you get Ready, Set and Go on this journey! Getting to the point where you have made your mind up that *I'm going to do things differently* takes courage. When you start to hear that voice inside clearly speak and you actually listen, that is all good! Congratulations, as you start your journey!

Peace Be With You

You may be running alone or physically with someone, but essentially you are running "alone" even if someone is behind you or in front of you. It's "your" run, and "your" commitment. So it's "your" time of peace. Don't be worried about anything at that time, just enjoy your run. You will know exactly what we are talking about, because you will get there and we will help you. This journey to fitness should always bring you a sense of peace. Enjoy the scenery of the locations you are running in for your routes. Enjoy watching the sunrise as you run. Don't try to rush through your run. As you take each step, let the peacefulness of what you are doing embark upon you. This is your time, so thank God for every breath you take, and enjoy the peace He has given you.

We Thank You

Take a bow and give yourself a pat on the back for taking the first step, which is picking up this book. We thank you from the bottom of our hearts for allowing us to share our journey with you. We also want to thank you for realizing our intention is to inspire and empower everyone to be the best they can become. For some, running is not easy or their thing. At the end of the day if you can't run, do something to become more fit and find a way to **Move and Smell the Roses!**

Chapter 12

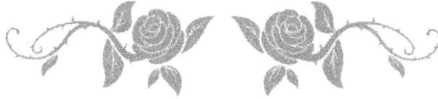

YOUR INCLUDED 90 DAY JOURNAL

Y ou will want to document your journey-days. We have included a 90-day journal for you in the back of this book. Commit to the first 90 days of using this journal and you will be amazed at your results. Having this journal to document your progress each day will be so helpful for you and is absolutely priceless.

Keep Up With Us And Who Else Is Running And "Smelling The Roses!"

This book is only the first step to us reaching out and helping others. We realize that after you read this book, you are going to need continued encouragement from others and to stay informed. Our website will provide you with those resources and more. Also, look for information on our website for our Run and Smell the Roses book signings, events and conferences.

Visit us:
www.runandsmelltheroses.com

Follow us:
Facebook: Run and Smell the Roses
Instagram: RunandSmelltheRoses
Twitter: @RunSmellRoses

Contact us:
runandsmelltheroses@mail.com

YOUR 90-DAY JOURNAL OF <u>YOUR</u> JOURNEY

HOW TO USE THIS JOURNAL

This journal allows plenty of creativity and free form expression. For the next 90 days use this journal to reflect on your feelings, thoughts, and accomplishments before, during, and after your run. Set your goals daily, weekly, and monthly using this journal.

DAY ONE
DATE:

DAY TWO
DATE:

DAY THREE
DATE:

_____

_____

_____

_____

_____

DAY FOUR
DATE:

_____

_____

_____

_____

_____

DAY FIVE
DATE:

_____

_____

_____

_____

_____

_____

DAY SIX
DATE:

_____

_____

_____

_____

_____

_____

DAY SEVEN
DATE:

DAY EIGHT
DATE:

DAY NINE
DATE:

DAY TEN
DATE:

<u>TIP</u>

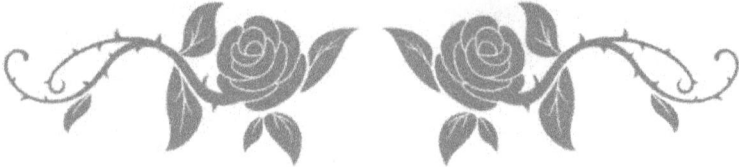

If you want to become a runner, start now.

Don't spend the rest of your life wondering if you can, there is no better time than today.

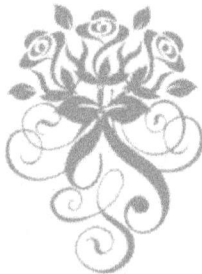

DAY ELEVEN
DATE:

_____

_____

_____

_____

_____

_____

DAY TWELVE
DATE:

_____

_____

_____

_____

_____

DAY THIRTEEN

DATE: _____

_____

_____

_____

_____

_____

DAY FOURTEEN

DATE: _____

_____

_____

_____

_____

_____

DAY FIFTEEN
DATE:

_____

_____

_____

_____

_____

DAY SIXTEEN
DATE:

_____

_____

_____

_____

_____

_____

DAY SEVENTEEN
DATE:

_____

DAY EIGHTEEN
DATE:

DAY NINETEEN
DATE:

_____

_____

_____

_____

_____

DAY TWENTY
DATE:

_____

_____

_____

_____

_____

Yolanda Diaz and Itarsha Payne

<u>TIP</u>

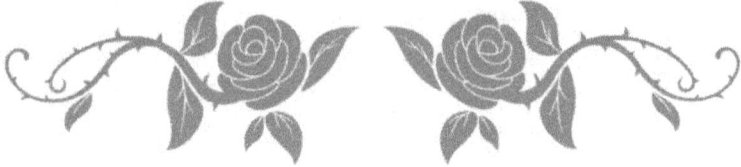

Everyone is an athlete underneath it all.

The only difference is that some of us work at it and some of us don't. Be the one to work on your inner athlete...run!

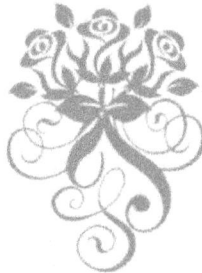

DAY TWENTY-ONE
DATE:

_____

_____

_____

_____

_____

DAY TWENTY-TWO
DATE:

_____

_____

_____

_____

_____

DAY TWENTY-THREE
DATE:

_____

_____

_____

_____

_____

_____

DAY TWENTY-FOUR
DATE:

_____

_____

_____

_____

_____

_____

DAY TWENTY-FIVE
DATE:

DAY TWENTY-SIX
DATE:

DAY TWENTY-SEVEN
DATE:

DAY TWENTY-EIGHT
DATE:

DAY TWENTY-NINE
DATE:

DAY THIRTY
DATE:

<u>TIP</u>

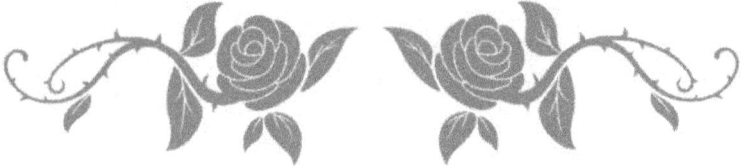

Running

....like anything you have to work at in life, you get out of it what you put in it.

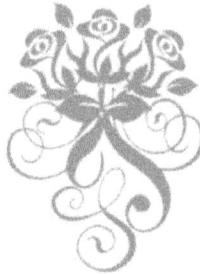

DAY THIRTY-ONE
DATE:

DAY THIRTY-TWO
DATE:

DAY THIRTY-THREE
DATE:

DAY THIRTY-FOUR
DATE:

DAY THIRTY-FIVE
DATE:

DAY THIRTY-SIX
DATE:

DAY THIRTY-SEVEN
DATE:

DAY THIRTY-EIGHT
DATE:

DAY THIRTY-NINE
DATE:

DAY FORTY
DATE:

<u>TIP</u>

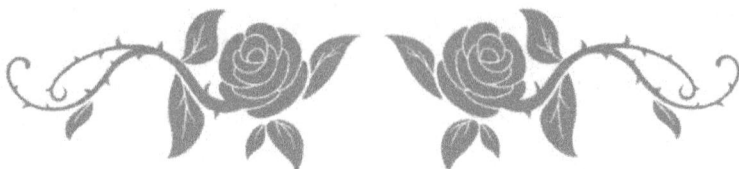

The sun can cause you to squint while running.

Wearing sunglasses during your run can reduce sunlight glare and squinting.

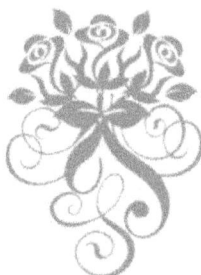

DAY FORTY-ONE
DATE:

DAY FORTY-TWO
DATE:

DAY FORTY-THREE
DATE: _____

_____

_____

_____

_____

_____

DAY FORTY-FOUR
DATE: _____

_____

_____

_____

_____

_____

DAY FORTY-FIVE
DATE:

DAY FORTY-SIX
DATE:

DAY FORTY-SEVEN
DATE:

DAY FORTY-EIGHT
DATE:

DAY FORTY-NINE
DATE:

DAY FIFTY
DATE:

TIP

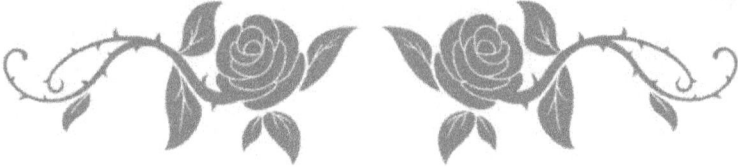

Find an internal rhythm.

A good way to do this is to listen to music while you run. You can even mouth the words. A standard 5-minute song will carry you through a half-mile or more.

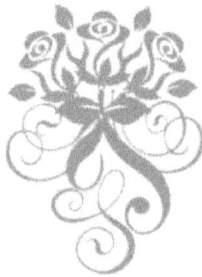

DAY FIFTY-ONE
DATE:

DAY FIFTY-TWO
DATE:

DAY FIFTY-THREE
DATE:

DAY FIFTY-FOUR
DATE:

DAY FIFTY-FIVE
DATE:

DAY FIFTY-SIX
DATE:

DAY FIFTY-SEVEN
DATE:

DAY FIFTY-EIGHT
DATE:

DAY FIFTY-NINE
DATE:

DAY SIXTY
DATE:

Yolanda Diaz and Itarsha Payne

TIP

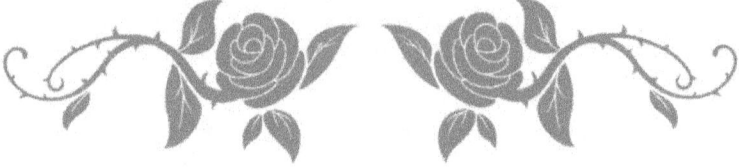

Don't forget your sunscreen!

The tip of your nose, the tops of your ears, hands, and your scalp are areas that you should pay special attention to when putting on sunscreen for your run.

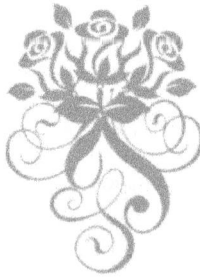

DAY SIXTY-ONE
DATE:

DAY SIXTY-TWO
DATE:

DAY SIXTY-THREE
DATE:

DAY SIXTY-FOUR
DATE:

DAY SIXTY-FIVE
DATE:

DAY SIXTY-SIX
DATE:

DAY SIXTY-SEVEN
DATE:

DAY SIXTY-EIGHT
DATE:

DAY SIXTY-NINE
DATE:

DAY SEVENTY
DATE:

<u>TIP</u>

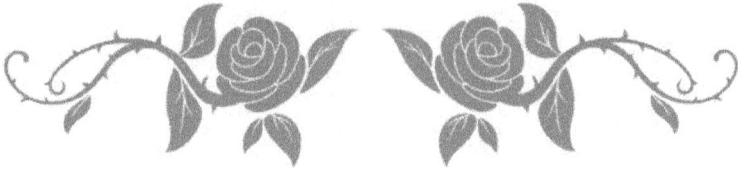

Remember... ... takes discipline to gain freedom,

take the time to be thankful while running.

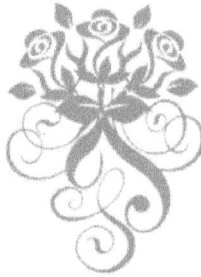

DAY SEVENTY-ONE
DATE:

DAY SEVENTY-TWO
DATE:

DAY SEVENTY-THREE
DATE:

DAY SEVENTY-FOUR
DATE:

DAY SEVENTY-FIVE
DATE:

DAY SEVENTY-SIX
DATE:

DAY SEVENTY-SEVEN
DATE:

DAY SEVENTY-EIGHT
DATE:

DAY SEVENTY-NINE
DATE:

DAY EIGHTY
DATE:

Yolanda Diaz and Itarsha Payne

TIP

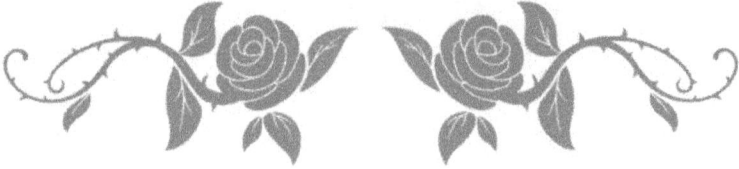

If you want to do something different

in your journal, write down what you saw while running, so you can document a voyage of exploration.

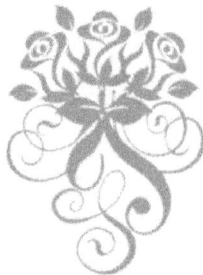

DAY EIGHTY-ONE
DATE:

DAY EIGHTY-TWO
DATE:

DAY EIGHTY-THREE
DATE:

DAY EIGHTY-FOUR
DATE:

DAY EIGHTY-FIVE
DATE:

DAY EIGHTY-SIX
DATE:

DAY EIGHTY-SEVEN
DATE:

DAY EIGHTY-EIGHT
DATE:

DAY EIGHTY-NINE
DATE:

DAY NINETY
DATE:

TIP

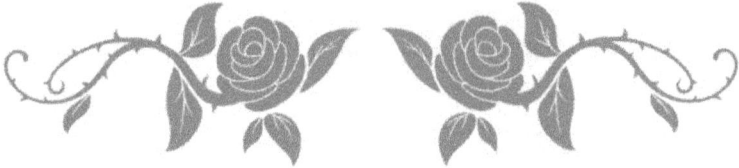

Sometimes run without a watch while running.

At times wearing a watch can create some unwanted pressure on yourself, which can take away the enjoyment. Once in a while run without being on a time limit and enjoy freedom!

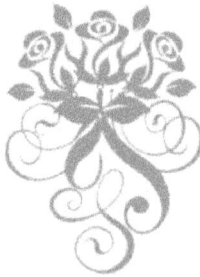

Research Sources:

Source: Wbur's Common Health
Website: comhealth.wbur.org
Article: Why are 4 out of 5 black women obese, overweight?
Author Rachel Zummerman, Nov. 29, 2012

Source: National Heart, Lung, Blood Institute
Website: nhlbi.nih.gov
Article: What are the Health Risks of Overweight & Obesity?
No author listed

Source: Women's Heart Foundation
Website: womensheart.org
Article: Women and Heart Disease Facts
No author listed

Yolanda Diaz

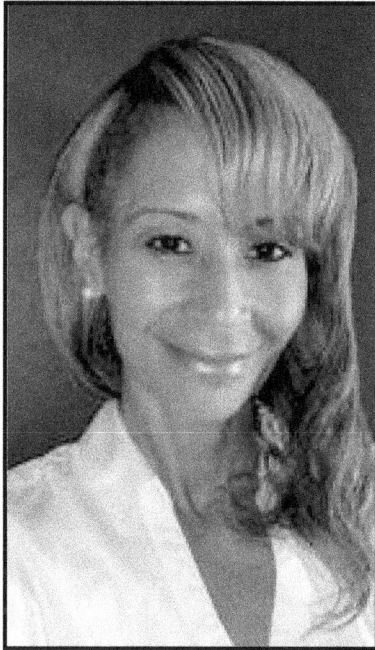

Yolanda Diaz began her professional career early on in the Hospitality Industry. She is a successful Sales and Marketing expert. Her proven abilities in maximizing and increasing revenue for hotels resulted in rapid advancement. Yolanda's dynamic personality and line of work in sales and marketing has always allowed her to express her enthusiasm, embracing and caring nature in making the "best" of anything even "better!" As a sales and meeting consultant, in addition to providing selling, marketing and meeting/event advice, she enjoys providing leadership skills and mentoring that leads to a positive change and culture. Yolanda has been running for over seven years and loves sharing how running has transformed her life. Her passion for wanting the best for herself and others crossed over to her wanting to be more fit and helping others become more fit and feel great! She relocated to North Carolina, in 1997 from Maryland. You may contact Yolanda at yolandarunandsmelltheroses@mail.com.

Itarsha Payne

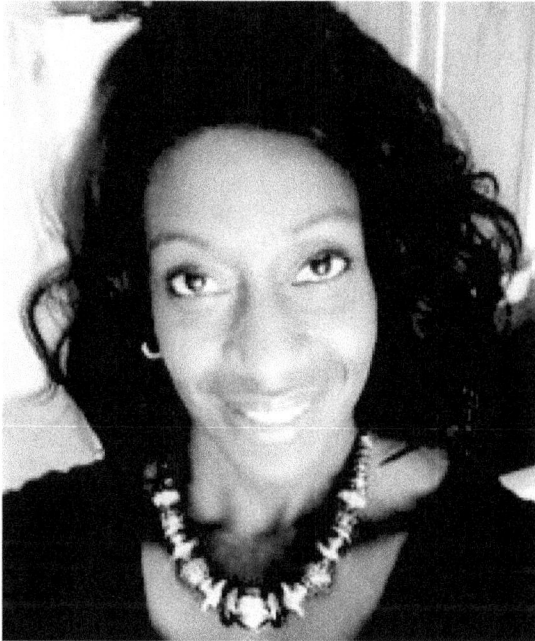

Itarsha Payne was born and raised in Brooklyn, New York. She left the hustle and bustle of city life behind and made North Carolina her home twenty-three years ago. Itarsha has a diverse and dynamic background, which extends from sales & marketing, to managing and operating multi-unit assets and real estate for almost fifteen years. Her multi-faceted background and skills, along with her entrepreneurial spirit, is what launched her into business ownership. Itarsha is co-owner and operator of Two Chicks And A Mop LLC and Two Chicks Fashions Boutique, both operating in Raleigh, North Carolina and surrounding areas. Both business enterprises are slated to expand outside North Carolina over the next five years. When she isn't busy running her two businesses, she's busy running, literally! Itarsha's love for running started over seven years ago and is still strong today. She contributes her love and dedication for running and living a healthy lifestyle to wanting to be the best version of herself that she can be, and to help others do the same. That love and passion for running is why she has shared her journey in hopes that you, too, will fall in love with running! Itarsha may be contacted via Facebook: Itarsha Payne or by email: itarsharunandsmelltheroses@mail.com

Thank You From The Publisher

Thank you for reading a book published by DCC Publishing, LLC. (dccpublishing@gmail.com). This book is available in Paperback and e-Book.

Please visit our website at www.runandsmelltheroses.com to find more on Yolanda Diaz and Itarsha Payne.

www.ingramcontent.com/pod-product-compliance
Lightning Source LLC
Chambersburg PA
CBHW072103020426
42334CB00017B/1616